WALKING
For
WEIGHT LOSS

Jago Holmes'

The Ultimate Walking Fitness & Weight Loss Program For Women

Quick Start Guide

Let's get started:

For anyone who wants to get started walking as quickly as possible

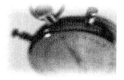

I'm already quite fit:

For anyone who already exercises regularly and wants a challenge

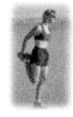

I want to know the details:

For anyone who's interested in the technical details of walking and weight loss

I need some motivation:

For anyone who needs a helping hand to get motivated

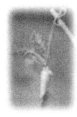

Hi There

A very warm welcome to '**Walking for Weight Loss**,' a weight loss program designed for women that want to lose weight and stay fit and active but don't necessarily want to be stuck in the gym or just go to a fitness class.

In this book, you'll discover how to use my unique 4 levels of walking to help you to lose weight, improve fitness and then, more importantly, maintain that weight loss.

Many people don't see the point of walking unless they have a dog to walk or if they've only got a very short distance to walk, but it's a fact that walking is a great and effective way to lose weight and stay in shape.

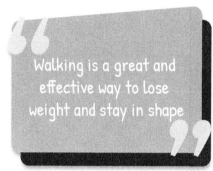

" Walking is a great and effective way to lose weight and stay in shape "

Walking is an exercise for everyone, whatever background they come from and no matter what they do for a living. And for those of you who have to sit in an office for 8 hours a day – it's even more important.

To get the most out of walking there are a few rules that you need to follow, if you get this right, you'll lose the most weight and see the quickest improvements in your fitness and energy levels. Here they are…

Set realistic goals!

Be prepared to make alterations to your lifestyle

Be consistent

Improve your diet

Make small but regular changes to your walks

Be patient and determined

But the best tip I can give you is to remember to enjoy it. The result is important, it's what you're aiming for after all, but the journey is also a big part of the process.

Finally, don't forget when you get to the shape and size that you want to be, you're going to need to maintain this new shape. And walking is the perfect solution, it's easy to fit into your lifestyle, you can do it anywhere, at any time. You can enjoy it with family and friends. And you don't need to spend a lot of money on equipment – an ideal solution.

I wish you the very best of luck and hope you enjoy every success with your weight loss journey.

To your health and fitness,

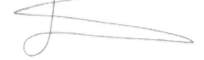

CONTENTS

WHY YOU SHOULD GO WALKING

Before we get into the details of setting your walking program, let's look at the benefits of walking.

Exercise through walking will give you an incredible boost to your overall health; including improved heart health and weight loss, as well as an improvement in your mental well-being – how you feel on a day-to-day basis.

Walking regularly can improve your sleep (insomnia affects 55% of us). It can also help improve your overall energy levels. We all get times when we lack energy, our lives are so busy – imagine if you could give yours a boost – without the sugary snacks.

You may believe that because walking isn't as high impact as some other forms of exercise, there aren't that many benefits compared to something like aerobics, however this is absolutely not the case.

Regular walking will help you to lose weight and can prevent disease and serious illness such as diabetes and arthritis.

Preventative:

Reduces the risk of:

- Coronary heart disease
- Stroke
- Osteoperosis
- Diabetes
- Arthritis
- May reduce risk of Alzheimers

Improves:

Reduces

- Cholesterol
- Body Fat

Benefits of walking

Social:

- Improves mental wellbeing
- Spend more time with family and friends
- Meet people (e.g. through walking clubs)

Personal:

- Saves money (e.g. petrol costs or bus fares)
- Helps the environment (less pollution)
- Reduces stress
- Improves sleep
- Raises energy levels

Walking regularly will improve your health, as well as reduce your risk of ill health. It will increase your overall muscle tone and bone density as well as lowering body fat levels.

If you commit to a regular walking schedule, then you'll start to feel much healthier and much less stressed.

Bearing in mind everything you've just read, why wouldn't you want to walk? If a miracle drug came along and promised all these benefits, you'd be taking it every day – **so let's get walking!**

Committing To Changing Your Lifestyle

You've proven that you're committed to making a change in your life and you've clearly been thinking about this – otherwise you wouldn't be reading this guide.

However, I know from experience that wanting to make a change and actually making that change is totally different.

So here are a few thoughts about starting off the right way and getting motivated...

Visualisation: The first thing I want you to do is to think about what this change to your lifestyle will look and feel like – fast forward six to twelve months ahead and imagine where you will be, what you'll be doing, how you'll look and how you'll feel as a result of your lifestyle change.

This might seem a bit strange, but visualising where you want to be is essential – how can you plan your journey if you don't know where the end is... sports stars use this all the time to help them.

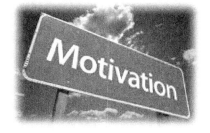

You shouldn't go off into the realms of fantasy, try not to think about magazine images, **think of an improved you**. Think of your friends commenting on 'how good you look these days', think about going to the shops and picking up clothes one size smaller, about feeling healthy and full of energy.

Remember these images; you can use them when it comes to the goal setting section further on.

Preparing for a change: Humans are programmed to take the easiest possible route in life, and we're also programmed to eat more than we need. So, to make a lifestyle change to get fitter and to lose weight may feel like you're working against your natural instincts at first. You need to prepare for this and be tough with yourself.

One of the best pieces of advice I ever had when starting out on changing my lifestyle was to 'never switch off'. You always have to be thinking about what exercise you need to do that day, and you always need to be thinking about what you're eating that day. **If you don't get tough with yourself, no one else will.**

YOU NEED TO TAKE RESPONSIBILITY FOR THE ACTIONS AND CHOICES YOU MAKE IN LIFE.

Dealing with setbacks: Everyone has setbacks, when you've invested so much into a change of lifestyle, as you will have done, any set back can seem overwhelming and enormous. You may be surprised by how emotional you get. However, don't let any setbacks defeat you. This is the time to get a supportive friend round or on the phone and have a good natter about what's on your mind. It's time to remember how much you achieved so far.

The main thing is to follow the famous phrase 'Keep calm and carry on', don't let a setback throw out your whole program, if you have a bad day or even a bad week, remember the images of the future you and get back on track. If you get an injury or can't walk, then try swimming instead – do something else, even housework is quite good for fitness. Keep positive and you'll survive through the tough times.

Mind and Goal Setting

Whilst your main goal may be to lose weight, one of the biggest changes you will see even within a few days of starting your chosen walking schedule is a boost in confidence and self-esteem.

Regular exercise will give you a huge psychological boost as well as a physical boost.

There are unlikely to be huge physical differences in body fat levels over the initial days, but the effects of taking control and being in charge of your own destiny will lead you to feel amazing at the beginning of any weight loss program.

Generally speaking, if you've been gaining weight for any amount of time a number of things may have happened to you:

- You will have stopped looking at yourself… I mean really looking at yourself.
- You will have become less interested in the way you present yourself.
- You will have accepted the fact that you never have any energy and even simple tasks can feel like an effort.
- You will have forgotten how it feels to like the way you look and to love the way you look seems an impossibility.
- Your confidence levels will have dropped.
- You will have started to dislike yourself.
- You will have accepted that life dictates to you, you'll believe you have no control over your own destiny.

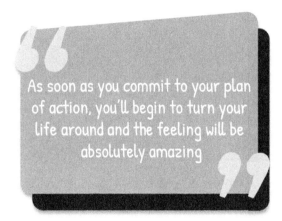

As negative as these factors are, they're all reversible, usually within a very short amount of time – I'm talking about days not weeks here.

Almost as soon as you commit to your plan of action, you'll begin to turn your life around and the feeling will be absolutely amazing.

YOU'LL decide the way you look, feel and act. YOU are in control. **You can do almost anything you want to do**.

Every journey starts with a single step; from simply going to the grocery store for a few things to trekking across Africa for the holiday of a lifetime. But two things always have to happen. First of all, you must decide what you're going to do and then second you must take action and do it.

Now in the case of nipping out to the grocery store, your plan might be as simple as writing a grocery list and making sure you have enough fuel in the tank to get there and back. If you were planning a trek across Africa however, there's going to have to be a lot more planning and organizing to do. Different things will be happening at different times and they all need to be planned to fit together correctly.

This is how it is with losing weight, the first thing you need to do is get a drink, pull up a chair, get a pen and paper ready and begin the process of setting down your goals. Once you've done this you need to write down how you're going to achieve these goals.

The Importance of Goal Setting

One of the most important steps in this process is to actually write your goals down. Your brain needs targets to aim for, this is the way we're conditioned. Most women have vague dreams and desires that they will probably never achieve because they never set them in motion. **A goal that excites, challenges, or inspires you is one that you are most likely to go on to achieve.**

You'll need to be determined and committed to achieve any weight loss goals and setting some structured short- and long-term goals will help to keep you motivated along the way.

There are two basic types of goals, process goals and outcome goals. It's important to set short-term objectives (process goals) on your way to achieving the big goal (outcome goal).

Let's take these in turn. Don't forget to have your pen and paper ready.

Process Goals:

These types of goals involve activities that help to improve your ability to achieve your outcome goals. Examples of process goals include:

- I will follow this training program closely.
- I will change my diet and only eat treat foods once a week.
- I will try to sleep at least 8 hours every night, etc.

Outcome Goals:

These goals relate to the finished product or end goal.

- I have lost 20lbs and I feel amazing.
- I have managed to fit back into my favorite jeans again.
- I really love the way I look and I'm so proud of myself for keeping going.
- I still walk regularly and monitor my weight to maintain the NEW me!

Ok, so these are the things you want, now you need to sit down and make a list of all the things that you'd like to accomplish through your training. Make two lists – one with process goals and when you want to achieve them by.

You should try to have some process goals to achieve every three months. The second list should have your outcome goals – where you want to be at the end of this process. Don't worry about whether they make any sense or not or are achievable at this stage, simply get your thoughts down on to paper…

Just brainstorm what you want to accomplish, we'll make sense of this next.

SMART Goals

When you've done this, we need to turn these goals in to SMART goals. The key to setting goals is to use the S.M.A.R.T. acronym.

The meaning of this is as follows:

S is for Specific	For example, if you want to get to a particular dress size for a special occasion, write down the exact dress size you want to wear and the exact date you want to wear it.
M is for Measurable	A measurable goal is one that you actually measure. For example, just stating you'll want to feel better isn't measurable, but if you say that now you feel like 5 out of 10 for wellness. A measurable goal would be to get to 7 out of 10 in 6 week's time.
A is for Achievable	If you set yourself unrealistic targets, you'll get demotivated when you don't achieve them. You should have a set of targets you can tick off as you travel towards your end goal. You'll feel boosted by achieving your goals along the way.
R is for Realistic	A realistic goal could be to drop 3 dress sizes, but this can't be achieved in only a few weeks. Dropping 3 dress sizes in 6 months could be realistic.
T is for Time Framed	You need to set yourself a timescale to achieve your goals, e.g. 'by my 30th birthday I am going to be a dress size 14'.

Another very important part of goal setting is to write them in the present tense (particularly for process goals) so they become more realistic in your own mind.

They have a much more powerful effect written in this way. By writing goals like this it's almost as though you're just recording what you've already achieved.

Example of a goal written in the future tense: I would like to be able to go swimming and feel happy about the way I look in my swimming costume in 6 week's time.

Not bad...

♦ It's specific – feel happy about the way I look in my bathing suit.
♦ It's measurable if we use our scale of 1 – 10 of happiness to record how we feel now and then again in 6 week's time.
♦ It's achievable depending on how it looks now.

- It's realistic.
- It's time framed – this is going to happen in 6 weeks from now.

But we can do better, how about this one…

I've just been swimming; it's been 6 weeks since I started my walking program and I feel amazing. I'm so proud of the way I look, slimmer and more toned. My wellbeing feels like an 8 out of 10. Not only that, but I could swim further, faster and I now have so much more energy. I'm really proud of what I've achieved.

This has much more emotion invested in it, and you can almost picture yourself feeling this way in 6 week's time, it links to the visualisation that I talked about earlier.

See if you can match your visualisation into some SMART goals written like this. This type of goal will help keep you motivated.

Another way to formalize a goal is to commit yourself financially. For example, once you've decided on a weight loss/dress/trouser size target, go out and actually buy some clothes in that size, but try on the larger size to see if the clothes suit you first.

By committing yourself financially to your goals, you are more likely to keep on track during the harder times of your training program.

One final but very important point you need to consider when setting goals is that they should be broken down in to smaller, more manageable chunks.

Here are some 'SMART' 6-week (process) goals:

"I have managed to follow the walking program this week"

"I have bought a new pair of jeans the next size down"

"I have changed the way I eat to a much healthier diet"

"I have lost ½ inch off my waist this week"

Good examples of long term (outcome) goals would be:

"I have completed a charity 10k run on dd/mm/yyyy. It was a great feeling finally realizing my goal after 6 months of training."

"Combined with my training and changes to my diet, I have lost 1 stone for my wedding anniversary on dd/mm/yyyy."

Rewrite your list of goals using our SMART chart and split them into short term (process) goals and longer term (outcome) goals.

You should then pin your goals up somewhere in your home – may be on your noticeboard or on your fridge – somewhere you'll keep reading them.

Well done! You've taken the first step towards a fitter and healthier lifestyle.

Your Workout Log

Another tool that you can use that goes hand in hand with your goal setting notes is to keep an activity log. It doesn't matter what you use to chart your progress, a diary, notebook, computer spread sheet, or anything, just do it.

Keep notes and record all the details about your training.

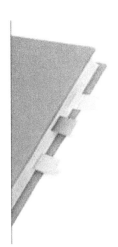

Some of the things you need to record are as follows:

- The date and time of day you do your walks.
- The distance or time that you have walked during that session.
- How you felt both physically and mentally, before, during and after the walk.
- You could also record your resting heart rate before you started and again straight afterwards.

If you use the same route over 2 or 3 different occasions and complete them in around about the same time, you should take your heart rate immediately after finishing each walk.

As you get fitter, you will in theory place less demand on your heart, therefore your heart rate should be slower (less beats per minute) on subsequent walks.

If you really want to go in to detail, you may want to include things like:

- The weather.
- The route you took.
- What you wore.
- Whether you felt any aches or pains.
- Your pre walk meal.

If you can track your heart rate, you could record your average and maximum heart rate throughout the course of your walk.

The main benefit of recording your walking workouts is to chart your progress. There are some blank workout logs for you to use at the end of the book.

Seeing how far you've come from your earlier workouts can really highlight the progress you've made, giving you a boost, especially on your down days. Also making a note of any aches and pains early on may help to prevent them developing into much more serious longer-term problems.

You will also find that committing these details to paper means that you're increasing the importance of this task in your life and programming your subconscious mind toward success.

Walking is lower impact than many other sports or activities however it still requires you to use the muscles in your body to generate movement and create stability that help to improve your balance and co-ordination.

When you move, your muscles contract around the joints to create that movement. The more often you move, then the more often your muscles contract. The great news for us is that every time our muscles contract, they need fuel.

The fuel our muscles use is a combination of the fats and carbohydrates that we have stored in our bodies. So, in basic terms, **the more we move, then the more weight we'll lose**, because our body is burning through its fuel quicker.

Higher-intensity exercises such as running will burn off more calories, simply because muscles need to contract much faster and work harder, therefore requiring more fuel.

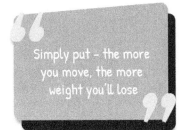

Simply put – the more you move, the more weight you'll lose

But here's the really clever part, most people can only run for so long before getting tired and having to stop, meaning they don't really burn off that many calories. However, most of us can keep going for much longer if we walk and *this is really the secret* behind 'Walking for Weight Loss.'

Walking is an aerobic activity, which means any type of exercise that causes the heart and lungs to work harder than in everyday life. Walking works the large muscles of the legs, and it also works many other smaller, deeper muscles which stabilize and support the joints to keep you upright and standing tall.

So, it's a great all-around form of exercise.

Walking & Weight Loss – The Facts

Clearly you want to lose weight and you're determined and ready to get started. You know you need to do some activity as well as improve your diet, so why not join a gym?

Many women think joining a gym is the quickest and easiest way to get fit, but this is far from true. You only need to look at gyms in early January and then again at the end of February to see that gyms don't work for most people.

The problem with joining a gym is that firstly you're going to need to pay a lot of money each month, and it's easier to join than to quit. Gym membership subscriptions are generally taken out of your bank account every month until your contract term expires, which is a fantastic business model for the gym because they know that once they've hooked customers in, they can then keep billing them until the customer ends the contract at the end of the term.

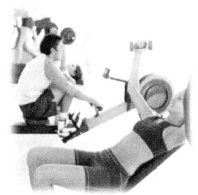

Unless you use the gym regularly and enjoy the experience, you won't get your money's worth and you may even feel like you've failed.

THE SECRET TO LOSING WEIGHT IS TO MAKE SURE THAT YOU TAKE PART IN EXERCISE THAT YOU ENJOY.

So, if you find it boring at the gym, it's unlikely to work for you. Why not try your local salsa dancing class, how about swimming, or even a local self-defence class instead. Pick something that gets you moving, motivated and suits your fitness levels. However, you can't say you don't enjoy something until you've tried it. So, keep an open mind and find a fun activity.

As we discussed in 'Goal setting' another key to success is to have a plan of action, something written down that you can look back on. It's important that you commit to your goals and targets, instead of simply keeping them in your head. It's even better if you tell someone else about your plans, perhaps a close friend who can help keep you on track.

The brilliant thing about walking is that it suits all abilities, its low impact (there's less risk of an injury), there's no special equipment needed, and IT WILL definitely **help you to lose weight if you commit to a regular plan.**

The key with walking is to be consistent. If you follow one of the walking plans in this manual and combine it with a healthy diet, you'll be amazed at the results. *Imagine how you would feel if you achieved your goals.* Every time you move around, you're walking and burning off calories. So, to lose weight you need to reduce your intake of calories a bit and increase the number of calories you burn off – it's as simple as that.

Imagine if you stopped using your TV remote control and switched channels manually; you could burn off half a pound of body fat in a year with just a simple change. Imagine the improvement if you made some bigger changes than that – perhaps getting off the bus one stop early and walking the rest of the way to work. The more time you move around then the more weight you'll lose.

How Many Calories Do You Burn While Walking?

Any type of movement or activity burns off calories, and the more challenging the exercise, then the more calories you'll burn off.

Exercises that involve moving the arms and legs at the same time will usually burn off more calories than doing either in isolation, which is another reason why walking is such a fantastic exercise because you can involve your arms at the same time as using the legs.

There are lots of ways to make walking more challenging (and therefore use up more calories) such as using hand weights, walking up hills or walking faster for short bursts of time (have a look at page 84 for more details about these)

In order to burn off 1lb of body fat, you need to use 3,500 calories more than you eat and drink.

This might seem like a huge number of calories, but if we take this over a week, then it's only *500 calories per day* (which is the equivalent to a fast-food burger or two slices of pizza)

REDUCING CALORIES IS BEST ACHIEVED THROUGH A COMBINATION OF BOTH DIET AND EXERCISE.

So, if you take out your favorite high fat/sugar snack each day at around 200 – 300kcals (e.g. choosing an Americano coffee instead of a Latte) AND you become more active then you will begin to see very quick changes indeed.

There are a number of factors involved in burning off calories through walking, such as how long you walk for, how much you weigh, how fast you walk, and your current fitness levels etc.

The chart below can be used as a guide, this shows how many calories an average person weighing around 168lbs would burn over the space of one hour working at different speeds.

These are only estimates, but the table below should help you to understand the link between the effort you make, or time spent walking, and the amount of calories you will burn off.

Time	3mph (brisk walk)		4mph (fast walk)	
	Distance	Calories	Distance	Calories
10 minutes	0.5 miles	54 kcals	0.65 miles	64 kcals
30 minutes	1.5 miles	163 kcals	2 miles	193 kcals
60 minutes	3 miles	327 kcals	4 miles	386 kcals

Measuring Weight Loss

If your aim is to lose weight or tone up, then you need to measure what is happening to your body and your overall shape to know if you're making progress.

It's very difficult to see the changes in the mirror alone, and *most of us have a distorted image of how we actually look anyway.*

Weighing scales can tell you how much you weigh overall but it probably won't accurately measure your progress.

Your weight is made up of bone, muscle, fat and water. It's not good to lose muscle, it's definitely not good to lose water but it is good to lose body fat if you are storing too much of it.

When dieting or changing eating habits, a lot of the initial weight loss is often due to a loss in the amount of water in your body. Once you start eating normally water and weight will be gained back immediately as your body doesn't like being dehydrated; it affects the body's internal water balance and can actually slow down the metabolism.

Losing muscle is not good either because this also slows down the metabolic rate.

LOSING BODY FAT IS THE GOAL OF ANY WEIGHT LOSS PROGRAM AND ITS SUCCESS CAN ONLY BE MEASURED BY THE AMOUNT OF FAT LOST, NOT OVERALL WEIGHT.

Here are the most effective methods of monitoring your progress:

Take a photo	• Take photos of yourself before you start. It's much easier to be objective when you look at a paper copy of yourself. Some people may find this a painful step, but it's a really important part to help you stay motivated. • Ideally you should take pictures wearing just your underwear, remember these are for your reference only. Taking shots from the front, back and both sides is the best way • Keep these photos near you and look at them regularly. This will keep you focused and drive you forward, particularly when you start to see changes
Use a piece of clothing	A pair of trousers, a skirt, some shorts, or a dress can be a good guide to your progress. Try them on every now and then to see if you're making progress. If they feel tight to begin with that's ideal
Use a tape measure	A simple tape measure found in sewing kits is probably one of the quickest and most practical ways of charting your progress. You should measure both around the hips and the waist to get a true indication of your progress
How you feel	Ask yourself regularly each week how you feel. Score this from one to ten, ten being fantastic and one being awful. Make a record of this figure in your diary
Get a body fat reading	If you have a gym membership, ask the staff there to take a body fat reading. The best and most reliable method of testing body fat levels and the loss of fat is by using skin fold calipers. All good gyms should be able to carry out this test for you quickly and reliably.

By taking measurements at regular intervals you are doing 2 things. Firstly, you can see whether your current efforts are having an effect, if they are, keep doing what you are doing, if not make some changes. For example, you might be able to increase the amount of activity you are doing. Secondly it maintains your awareness and helps to keep you focused on your goals and objectives.

When measuring around the waist, don't tense or pull in your tummy muscle, just stand relaxed.

When measuring your hips, stand with your feet together.

I suggest taking the measurement 2 or 3 times just to make sure that you've got it right.

Make sure that you can retake the measurement again in the same place the next time, so put the same amount of tension on the measuring tape.

Another sign of healthy weight loss and an active lifestyle are your skin, hair and nails. These virtually always look and feel better when you start to lose weight or become more active.

If you are still intent on judging your success by standing on a set of scales each week, bear in mind that you're only getting part of the picture.

The best way to monitor your progress is to use a combination of methods and never just rely on weighing scales alone.

How to Change Your Diet to Lose Weight

THE KEY TO LOSING WEIGHT AS FAST AS POSSIBLE IS TO MAKE SMALL CHANGES TO YOUR DIET.

If your weight is currently static (you're not gaining or losing weight) then you'll see the best results by cutting out between 200 – 300kcals a day. This is easily done by sacrificing any of your higher calorific treats such as a latte, cookie, bag of potato chips, candy bar etc.

If your diet doesn't contain any of these types of foods, then you'll need to look a little deeper and cut down on any excess fats or sugars you may use.

If you're currently gaining weight, then you'll need to reduce your calories by more than this and adopt a new approach to eating.

Did you know that 1 in 3 women who diet end up weighing more than when they first started.

The main reason for this is because they choose crash diets which promise rapid weight loss, but ultimately lead to food deprivation. The dieter quickly becomes tired of the starvation diet and then binges on all of the forbidden foods. Any weight lost is quickly regained.

If you want lasting results, you must stay well clear from any diet that

- *Promises unrealistic weight loss.*
- Is based on an off the wall or unbalanced eating program.
- Tells you to eat certain amounts of some foods (like meat) in unlimited quantities, but prohibits the consumption of others (like bread or fruits).

These diets are unhealthy because they lack basic nutrients and can easily lead to eating disorders.

Here are the 6 key steps for a balanced diet:

Eat 5 smaller meals throughout the day	Don't' skip meals, especially breakfast and try not to leave your stomach empty for long periods, instead eat small, frequent meals that are easier to digest. Eat in moderation from all food groups (meats, fruits, veg, etc)
Reduce your fat intake	Fat is the highest source of calories (9 calories per 1 gram). Avoid eating fried foods, instead boil or bake foods after removing any visible fat. Avoid cakes, pastries and pies, mayonnaise, cream and dressings. Choose low fat dairy products
Reduce the amount of sugar you eat	Sugar is added to many processed, pre-packaged foods. If you can't get by without it, try to have no more than 2 teaspoons of sugar a day, preferably brown sugar
Eat plenty of fiber	Fiber helps to cleanse the digestive system and gives a feeling of fullness in the stomach which can reduce appetite. Eat wholemeal bread instead of white
Eat less salt	Don't put extra salt in your food and don't keep it on the table when eating. Avoid foods with a very high salt content, like tinned or processed food or sauces
Keep a food diary	If you record everything you eat or drink for a week and then read it, you will realize a lot about your eating habits from doing this and maybe find where there are some hidden calories

It's very common to underestimate how much food we eat. Many people consume a lot more calories than they realise and end up feeling frustrated about not being able to lose weight.

They often blame their bad metabolism or their family genes, but the truth is that **what they really need to do is to reduce their portion sizes.**

Easy Option Diet

To have a healthy and rounded diet, you should ideally choose a food from each list to make a meal.

- Eat a protein with a carbohydrate and a portion of vegetables.
- Each nutrient should be of equal size, about the amount you can hold in a cupped hand.

The lists don't include every possible option but are as follows:

Carbohydrates	Proteins	Vegetables
Whole wheat pasta	Skinless Chicken or Turkey	Green leafy vegetables
Butternut squash	Fish – not battered or fried	Carrots
Brown rice	Shellfish	Broccoli
Baked or boiled potato	Egg whites	Tomatoes
Oats	Cottage cheese	Onions
Whole wheat bread	Low fat yoghurt	Mushrooms
Corn	Lean beef	Peppers
Barley or couscous	Semi or skimmed milk	Celery
Bulgar wheat	Tofu	Aubergine
Sweet potatoes	Quorn	Cauliflower
Quinoa	Beans and pulses	Peas

An example meal might be brown rice, chicken (baked in foil) and steamed broccoli. An example breakfast might be porridge with a homemade sugar free fruit smoothie.

The key to changing your eating habits for the long term is to phase all these changes in slowly over a couple of months. Try to get the hang of maybe just drinking water in week 1. Then in week 2 you might decide to cut out pies, pastries and puddings and so on.

REMEMBER THIS IS A LIFE CHANGING EATING PLAN WHICH WILL KEEP YOU HEALTHY WELL IN TO OLD AGE.

Drink plenty of Water: Aim to drink at least 2 litres of fresh water a day. Tip – Fill a 2 litre bottle and drink from that bottle all day. Doing this ensures that you know how much you have drunk. Water helps to cleanse the system and maintain hydration.

Eat more fruit and vegetables: You should aim to eat at least 5 portions of fresh fruit and vegetables each day. This total can include frozen and tinned in water or juice as opposed to sweetened syrup. Tip – **Always keep a fruit bowl handy and full of fruit favorites**.

Think natural: Try to eat foods that are as close to their natural state as possible with minimum processing. Tip – Get into the habit of examining food labels, generally speaking the fewer ingredients added the closer it will be to its natural state.

Always eat breakfast: After a night of sleep the metabolism slows right down – as you've not digested any food. Eating breakfast will kick-start the metabolism for the day and help you lose more weight. Tip – Try a slice of toast with a thin spreading of no added sugar fruit spread immediately after waking.

Many women complain of a sickly feeling after eating in the morning, but this will disappear when the body is trained in to accepting breakfast.

No food is a sin: By cutting out certain foods from your diet your body will crave them even more. Choose one treat food and one or two days a week to have it and stick to this. Most *sin* foods are high in calories but low in nutritious bulk therefore you don't feel full after eating and as a result eat more total calories as well as those calories found in the *sin* foods.

> The key to changing your eating habits for the long term is to phase all these changes in slowly over a few months.

Eat more wholegrain products: Eating wholegrain foods will give your diet the maximum natural goodness as possible, you will feel fuller after eating and your food will be digested more easily. Tip – As a tasty nutritious snack why not try toasted wholemeal muffins with a little low-fat spread or for main meals use brown rice as the base.

Try to find healthy alternatives: Look at your favorite meals and try to find better ways of preparing them. Search for healthier take away options and less fatty restaurant foods. Tip – Fries can be replaced by oven baked potato wedges cooked in olive oil.

Experiment with foods: Try different foods - you might enjoy them.

Eating a variety of foods will ensure you get a variety of vitamins and nutrients, which will make you feel healthier. Tip – During your weekly shop aim to buy one new nutritious item and try one new recipe or meal each week.

Cut down on saturated fats: By reducing your intake of saturated fats you are doing one of the single most beneficial things to improve your health. Tip – Aim to become more aware of the fat content of foods and try to buy foods with minimal amounts of or no saturated fats in the ingredient listings.

Don't listen to people who put you down: Decide on your goals and write them down.

Don't listen to people who put you down or get in the way of you achieving your goals. Tip – Find a picture of the way you would like to look and keep this on display, be realistic but be determined.

We have the power to change and shape our bodies in incredible ways.

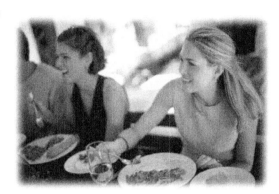

REMEMBER FAILURE IS NOT FALLING DOWN ITS STAYING DOWN.

Eating Out

Very often socialising with friends or family involves food, eating out at restaurants, the local pub or just a simple take away. **An effective eating plan should allow for the occasional treat and luxury.**

My advice is to eat out or have a take-out only once a week and less if possible. In my experience eating out more often than this is counter-productive and can lead to either an increase in body fat or a plateau where no progress is made.

Eating out doesn't have to spell disaster for your weight loss plans.

If you have a few meals out one week you should either increase your activity levels to compensate or accept that this week will be a bad one and that you might gain some weight.

When embarking on any program to change your health and the way you look and feel, it is inevitable that there will be times when you can't eat all the right things all the right times. The following list will give you some guidance on how you can make eating out as healthy and as hassle free as possible.

Ordering:

- Choose fresh fruit or bread starters (not garlic bread)
- Ask for vegetables that are unglazed with butter.

- Order burgers without cheese, special sauces or mayonnaise.

- Choose a vegetable or fish pizza with reduced cheese.

- Choose fish, chicken or turkey as opposed to red meat.

- Ask for reduced amounts of sauces with your meal.

Alternatives:

- Try boiled rice instead of fried.

- Order a side salad or vegetables instead of fries.

- If it's a salad bar choose fresh greens instead of bacon bits, potato salad or coleslaw.

- Share a dessert, you will consume 50% less calories.

- Choose ice cream instead of double cream.

Avoid:

- Fast food take outs as they are some of the highest fat foods around – avoid these.

- Avoid foods described as korma, creamy sauce, coconut or fried.

- Leave the mayo in the jar, each dollop contains around 100kcals.

- Don't add salt at the table, chefs often add salt to meals, so you won't need any extra.

How To Walk

Your Walking Gait

'Gait' is a term for the way you walk. You may think we all walk in the same way but there are subtle but important differences. It's very important that you have the right footwear for your gait. By choosing the right training shoes you can avoid placing a strain on the muscles and joints of the body over the course of your walking.

You can find out what your gait is by carrying out a few simple assessments. Another term used when talking about gait is 'pronation' – this is the way that the lower legs absorb shock, it's the movement of the foot from when your heel strikes the ground to the point where your big toe leaves the ground, or the amount of rolling your foot does towards the inside or instep of the foot.

There are three ways that you can learn how your foot lands and leaves the floor:

1. Look at Your Shoes

Have a look at the soles of the shoes you wear most often. If most of the wear is on the outside or outstep of the sole, you will generally tend to **under pronate**, but if the wear is more towards the inside or the instep of the sole, you are probably an **overpronator**.

If the wear appears evenly distributed over the sole, then the chances are you have a 'neutral' walking gait.

2. The Wet Foot Test

Wet the sole of your bare foot and walk on something that will clearly show a footprint. Some coloured paper, a tiled floor or even floorboards should be able to leave a mark that you can look at, which will show you how your foot lands.

3. The Treadmill Test

Specialized analysis equipment can also be used to find out your gait and this is probably the most reliable method. Most good running stores now have this technology free for you to use. During the test, your footprint is actually checked using a treadmill or a sensored pad, the tester can then see where the foot impact is the greatest and accurately predict your type of pronation.

Foot arches:

The marks left by the 'Wet Foot Test' will show you whether you have sunken (low) arches, neutral arches or raised arches which all indicate a certain type of foot pronation.

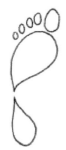 **Raised arches** – Indicate that your feet under-pronate when walking

If your footprint looks like this, you are an under pronator and have a high arched foot. Your footprint will leave a very thin band on the lateral side (outside of the foot) or none, between the heel and forefoot. This is because under pronators mainly only use their heels downhill. This curved, highly arched foot does not pronate sufficiently and requires a lot of cushioning.

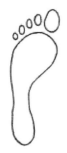 Neutral arches – This footfall is ideal for walking

If your print looks like this, you have a normal foot plant and are a neutral walker. A normal foot usually leaves approximately half the footprint - the lateral (outside) part.

Low arches – Indicates over-pronation because there is only a small amount of support stopping your foot rolling inwards.

If your print looks like this and your foot leaves a print of the whole of the foot, you have a flatter foot because the arch collapses through the foot motion. The foot strikes at the heel and rolls inwards excessively - this is over-pronation. If you are a serious over-pronator and do not wear the correct shoes, then you are much more likely to suffer from muscle and joint strains (especially knee and hip strains) when walking.

3 Types of Pronation:

Under-pronation (supination):

If you are an **under-pronator**, you will be in the minority, as this is the least common type of running gait. This style involves pushing off from the outside of the foot and will require more support on the outside of your shoes.

Neutral pronation:

This is the most desirable type of pronation where the foot plant lands on the outside of the heel and rolls inward slightly to absorb shock whilst moving off the big toe.

Over-pronation:

This is the most usual type of walking gait, nearly 70% of the population have this type of gait. If you over-pronate, your foot will land on the outer edge of the heel which flattens the arch as the foot strikes the ground and as the footstep progresses to push off it rolls excessively towards the instep.

This type of gait usually needs supports for the inside or instep of the shoe. These supports can be found quite widely on the high street, usually in a large chemist shop. You may want to get the opinion of a podiatrist if you're still unsure of what type of gait you have, or if you experience any soreness or stiffness in your legs after walking.

Most of the time our gait isn't important and we can cope quite well.

However, when you start to exercise regularly and for longer distances then **there is a risk of developing injuries due to the way you walk.**

Understanding your gait and getting the right shoes and supports can help prevent any injuries.

If you do have an injury, you should get it checked out by a doctor or physiotherapist straight away.

Picking The Right Shoes:

There is no such thing as the perfect walking shoe because everyone has different needs as a walker. The key factors to consider when choosing your shoes should be your gait, body weight, shape and width of your foot, the surfaces you walk on and how often you walk.

Having the correct fit is the most important part of the equation to get right when choosing your footwear and clothing. This is not only to achieve maximum performance, but also to avoid blistering and more serious injuries.

Training shoes are usually split in to three basic categories – cushioned, support and control.

Cushioned Shoes:

These shoes are for under-pronators. Walkers requiring cushioned shoes often walk more on their toes and have a raised arch. These training shoes provide little stability but are softer under foot and more cushioned.

Support Shoes:

Suitable for neutral walkers, support shoes are usually best for those with a 'regular' or neutral foot plant. Support shoes usually combine good cushioning with lightweight support features on the medial (inner) side of the shoe in order to limit excessive inward rolling of the foot.

Control Shoes:

Suitable for the more serious over-pronators and also for heavier walkers. Serious overpronators usually have a flatter foot as their arch collapses through the foot strike. These shoes are generally heavier and combine cushioning with extra support to provide essential protection which reduces the risk of injury.

Do I Need New Shoes?

Decide if you need to buy new shoes based on how old and how many miles your shoes have covered. Make sure that they aren't too old and still have cushioning present in the sole which helps to maximize the absorption of the impact of your stride and that they suit your walking gait.

The mid-soles of many training shoes break down at around 350 - 400 miles and they will offer little or no protection after that.

IT'S IMPORTANT TO KEEP IN MIND THAT TRAINING SHOES PROVIDE THE FIRST LINE OF DEFENCE AGAINST A POTENTIAL INJURY.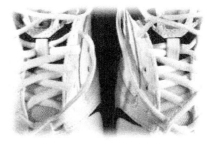

A good idea is to buy two pairs of the same training shoes and then alternate their use each training day. This increases the life expectancy of each pair. Try not to get too hung up on the colour or the look of your shoes, you should choose the right ones for your feet before anything else.

A specialist walking or running shop may be the best place to go if you're not sure what shoes to choose. Try on shoes later in the day when your feet have swollen to their full size and take the socks you normally use when exercising with you.

The shoes need to mould to the shape of your feet so they should be a snug fit at the sides and across the top. **Good training shoes tend to be as light weight as possible** at the same time as offering the maximum amount of support for your foot and gait type.

Pick the right shoe size: There should be no movement or slippage at the heel and check that your toes are not crushed into the toe box at the front of the shoe. Your foot can expand when walking longer distances, so you might need a shoe size a little bigger.

The usual recommendation is to allow half an inch or a thumb width of room from the front of your running shoe to the end of the longest toe. This extra room in the toe box helps avoid painful sore toes and nasty black toenails.

Walking surface: Your shoe needs to have the correct sole type for the surface you'll mainly be walking on. Road shoes have a shallow hard-wearing tread. Off road shoes require a tread with deep enough lugs for grip whilst being durable enough not to wear out on roads.

Broad or narrow foot: You need to find shoes that fit the width of your foot as well as the length. Most brands are built on a standard D width fitting, some are broader and some narrower than normal, so try a few different styles to find the best fit for you.

Buy shoes suitable for your gender: Men and women's feet vary in shape and size; it's essential to make sure that you buy a shoe specific to your gender.

Female feet are narrower, particularly around the heel and men's feet tend to be broader.

If you do decide to buy new shoes, a really important thing to **remember is to wear them in before you go out on a long walk.** Wear them round the house for an hour each day for a couple of weeks and then try them out for a short walk before putting them into regular use.

Shoe Care:

- Wear your training shoes only for your walking exercise sessions, they will last much longer.
- Do not machine wash or tumble dry your training shoes. If your shoes become dirty, hand wash them with commercial shoe care products.
- When your shoes become wet, stick bundled up newspaper inside to accelerate the drying time and help them to keep their shape.

Socks: Socks are also are a very important factor to consider as your feet will be subjected to constant movement, friction and rubbing.

You should buy a couple of good quality, specialized walking or running synthetic blend socks, which will wick sweat away from the skin and allow your feet to breathe.

Monitoring Intensity

Walking is a very enjoyable activity and you can increase or decrease the difficulty level in a number of ways.

It shouldn't be a chore that you hate doing or a punishment that you need to suffer in order to help you to lose weight or get fitter.

However, in order to get the results you want, you need to set some structure to your walking and you can achieve this by following the walking programs in this training manual which are progressive walking programs that allow you to improve consistently without risking overuse injuries or illness.

By ticking off goals and mini targets along the journey, you will start to feel a sense of accomplishment and satisfaction from your efforts.

The opposite is also true, without doing this you can quickly become de-motivated and bored with your training.

GETTING THE RIGHT INTENSITY IS VITALLY IMPORTANT.

If you don't work hard enough, you'll never make any real progress. During your walks you'll need to perform some sessions at different intensities to enable you to make steady and constant progress.

Walking longer distances at a comfortable pace will allow you to improve your endurance, and doing shorter walks at higher levels of intensity will build up leg strength and improve your body's ability to remove lactic acid from the muscles much faster, allowing you to work harder for longer. This is ideal if your walks contain any hills or gradients.

Aerobic Exercise: The American College of Sports Medicine (ACSM) defines aerobic exercise as '*any activity that uses large muscle groups, can be maintained continuously, and is rhythmic in nature.*'

This type of exercise causes the heart and lungs to work harder than in everyday life.

Aerobic exercise basically means exercising in the aerobic training zone (a level at which your heart beats faster than in normal life and for a prolonged period of time).

At this level of difficulty, you should still be able to hold a conversation with someone quite easily. Once your speed or distance begins to increase so that you are no longer able to talk then you are moving past the aerobic threshold and towards anaerobic training (a level of training whereby the demand for oxygen from the muscles is far greater than that being supplied to them).

Aerobic (or endurance) training improves the endurance of your heart and lungs by increasing both the amount of blood that the heart can pump and your muscle's ability to extract oxygen from that blood.

ANY WALKING PROGRAM SHOULD BE DESIGNED TO IMPROVE YOUR CARDIOVASCULAR ENDURANCE, MUST OVERLOAD YOUR HEART AND LUNGS AND IMPROVE YOUR MUSCLE'S ABILITY TO UTILIZE OXYGEN EFFICIENTLY.

There are two methods of monitoring your exercise intensity, Target Heart Rate and Perceived Exertion. These are explained next...

Target Heart Rate Zones: To get the most cardiovascular benefits from your workout, it is recommended to exercise within a certain intensity range.

In order to arrive at a given intensity range for the level of effort you are training at, it's necessary to have a starting point. A standard way to measure this is to estimate your maximum heart rate (Max HR) and use this as a starting point.

To find out your Max HR simply subtract your age from 220.

For example, if you are 30 years old, your predicted maximum heart rate per minute is 190 (this is calculated as follows: 220 - 30 = 190). Your target heart rate is a percentage of this maximum heart rate, shown in the chart below.

Target Heart Rates will vary for each individual depending on age, current level of conditioning, and personal fitness goals and running objectives.

However, for the bulk of your own training, your exercising heart rate should range between 50% to 70% of your maximum heart rate.

You can use the following chart to determine your predicted Target Heart Rate.

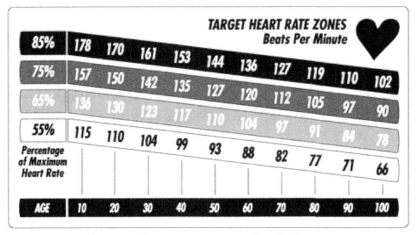

The heart rate zones as shown above are given the following meanings: -

55% (50 – 60%) - Aerobic Beginners Zone

65% (60 – 70%) - Fat Burning Zone

75% (70 – 80%) - Aerobic Fitness Zone

85% (80 – 90%) - Peak Performance Zone

Ideally you want to be working generally within these parameters, so using our example above, the aerobic heart rate training zone range for a 30-year-old is 95 to 171, which is 50% - 90% of 190 (Max HR).

To accurately measure your heart rate during exercise you'll need to purchase a heart rate monitor.

If this sounds a little too technical for you then don't worry, there is a much easier way of monitoring the intensity of your training called the *rate of perceived exertion or RPE scale.*

Rate of Perceived Exertion: (RPE) is one of the easiest ways to monitor exercise intensity. By using the RPE scale, you can continually assess your level of intensity during your workouts and ensure you are working at a level of effort or intensity that is comfortable and appropriate for you.

You can use the RPE scale on its own or with a heart rate monitor.

An increase in exercise intensity will always lead to an increase and elevation in your heart rate and consequently your rate of perceived exertion (how difficult you find it).

There are a number of ways of interpreting the RPE scale, but I like to use the scale below as I feel this is more easily understood than other versions that use numbers up to 20 to gauge intensity.

RPE SCALE	
1	Don't feel anything
2	Not at all challenging
3	Starting to feel something
4	Notice some effort
5	Feeling moderately challenging
6	Getting harder
7	Feeling quite hard
8	Feels very hard
9	Becoming very, very hard
10	That's it, you absolutely have to give up NOW!

Using the RPE scale as above, the recommended range during the majority of your training walks is between 5 (moderate) and 7 (feeling quite hard).

Some training techniques will obviously require you to work harder than this and these are outlined in the training techniques section.

Walking Technique:

One of the most important things you need to consider when walking is how your body moves when you walk. This may sound strange because you've been walking all your life. But it's different now that you're walking for a purpose.

With this walking program you will lose weight AND improve your posture at the same time. But if you're not walking correctly this could be placing stress on supporting and stabilising muscles which are not used to working this way.

Let's start with the correct posture. **Adopting a good posture will help you to conserve energy and walk faster** without putting stress on the lower back, hips, knees and ankles.

10 Point Posture Check:

Stand in front of a mirror so you can see your full-length reflection. Place your feet about hip width apart with your arms hanging relaxed down by your sides. Stand as you normally would do for a moment and go through the list below, give yourself a tick if you're doing any of these naturally...

☐	1.	Stand up tall and straight
☐	2.	Don't arch your back, imagine there's a piece of thread running through your body from your feet up through to the top of your head. Think about the thread being pulled tight, so that your head is held high
☐	3.	Don't lean in any direction either forwards, backwards or to one side or another.
☐	4.	Keep your head up without jutting out your chin, looking forwards without moving up or down or to the left or right.
☐	5.	Keep your chin up, not tucked on to your chest.
☐	6.	Stand with your chest lifted and forward, gently squeezing the shoulder blades together can help with this.
☐	7.	Your shoulders should be relaxed to reduce tension and allowed to rest back and down, again a gentle squeeze of the shoulder blades can help to promote this.
☐	8.	Keep your shoulders level
☐	9.	Pull your tummy muscles in. Try to imagine you have a thread running through your back and attached to your belly button, now imagine pulling on that thread to pull your belly button backwards towards your spine.
☐	10.	Tip your hips back very slightly and tuck your buttocks in and squeeze gently. It can sometimes be useful to imagine that you are trying to hold a coin between the buttocks as this helps to promote the gentle squeezing movement.

How many ticks did you get?

Any that you didn't get right try and adjust now, then stand for a couple of minutes in this new position.

Whilst you're doing this, be aware of how it feels. It may feel strange at first.

Take a few moments to get to grips with how your body feels when standing properly.

When you start your walks, this is something you should focus on. Doing this means that you'll not only be losing weight, but also working on correcting poor posture and body alignment.

If you spend a lot of time at a desk for work, it's very likely that your posture will be slouched over. It's really important to try and correct this or you could end up with lots of back pain, perhaps even suffering long term damage.

Now for the hard part, maintaining your posture at the same time as moving your legs and arms.

Leg movement: When walking you should use a heel to toe action. This means that the heel hits the ground first and then you roll forwards on to the toes, just before you push off again from the toes.

You should land each footstep on to the heel of the foot and then push off again from the toes.

This pattern of movement continues regardless of what terrain or surface you are walking on.

Remember at the same time as doing this with your feet you're also maintaining good posture, so your tummy muscles are pulled in, your shoulders are back and relaxed and your chest is lifted and open.

You'll be walking with your head held high... and a smile on your face!!

Arm movement: Bringing the arms in to play can help to increase the intensity of your workouts and help you to burn up to 10% more calories. Keep your arms almost straight and by your sides, they should move straight forwards and backwards in time with your feet.

Don't clench your hands to make a fist, keep the fingers relaxed, it's ok to curl the fingers, just don't clench as this can lead to an increase in blood pressure and a rise in tension.

When we step forwards, we use our arms to counterbalance our core muscles and we can increase speed and intensity by adding in extra arm movement. With every step you take, the opposite arm should move forwards.

Try to ensure that your arms move forwards and backwards by your sides, **not diagonally across your body.**

Don't exaggerate the movement so the arms come up higher than the chest in front or too high backwards. Try not to stride out too far especially in the early stages of the program or at the beginning of a walking session, as you're much more likely to pull a muscle or cause yourself other injuries.

If you want to go faster at this stage, then you should use smaller, quicker steps.

The Different Levels of Walking

Level 1 Walking:

Let's look at the different levels of walking in detail now. The pictures below show all the points we've just discussed clearly.

The first of our 4 different levels of walking is level 1 and I would describe this speed as strolling.

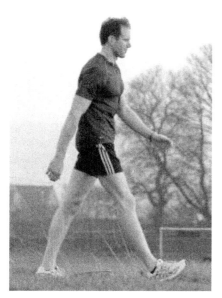 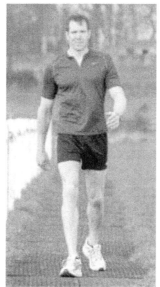 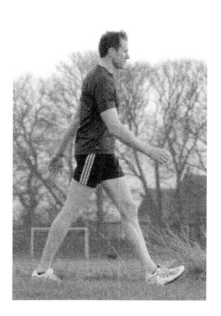

Here's a quick recap of how it should be done...

When walking you should use a heel to toe action. This means that the heel hits the ground first and then you roll forwards on to the toes, just before you push off again from the toes.

Remember at the same time as doing this with your feet you're also maintaining good posture, so your tummy muscles are pulled in, your shoulders are back and relaxed and your chest is lifted and open.

Keep your arms almost straight and by your sides, they should move straight forwards and backwards in time with your feet.

Don't clench your hands to make a fist, keep the fingers relaxed

There are 3 other levels of walking, level 2, level 3 and level 4. We'll take a look at all of these individually in turn now...

Level 2 Walking:

I like to think of this level of walking as that of being in a rush to get somewhere.

Imagine that you're running late for a bus, or a train and you need to get there quickly, this is the type of speed that you'll be walking at here.

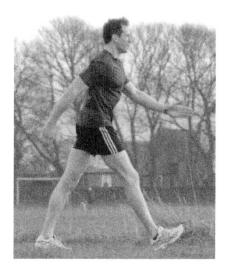 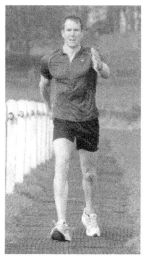 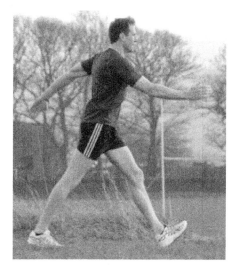

It's a very good starting point for beginners as it's challenging but not as intense as levels 3 and 4.

Here's how to do it...

Check your posture first - keep your head up, your shoulders back, pull in your tummy muscles and remember the idea of the string running up through your body pulling taut. Now on to the action itself...

The elbows should be bent only slightly and fixed in this position with your arms swinging from the shoulders not the elbows.

Remember to keep the arm swing straight forwards and backwards instead of across the body. They should not cross the body as this twists the hips, placing more stress on the core muscles. Don't clench your hands, simply relax the fingers in a curled or straight position.

The leg stride should be powerful and controlled with the heel hitting the ground first and rolling through on to and then off the toes.

Point the toes out to the sides slightly more than when just strolling (level 1).

You should walk as if in a rush, not the fastest speed you can go at but quicker than level 1.

Level 3 Walking:

This level of walking is much more aggressive and purposeful than the other two levels we've covered so far and there are distinct differences involved here.

Level 3 walking challenges the heart and lungs to a greater extent than previous levels and due to the faster speed and increased movement in the arms, **you'll burn off more calories and become fitter.**

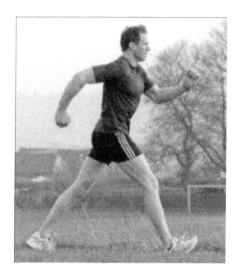 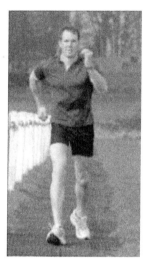 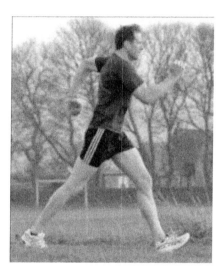

This is how to do it...

Check your posture first - keep your head up, your shoulders back, pull in your tummy muscles and remember the idea of the thread running up through your body pulling taut.

The elbows should be bent to approximately 90 degrees and fixed in this position. The swing is still generated from the shoulders but because the arms are bent, they are shorter and can be moved much faster which will also increase the speed in leg movement.

Keep the arms close into the body so they act as pistons which can be moved faster to generate more power and speed. The shoulders still need to be relaxed, back and down to reduce any tightness or tension build up caused by the movement and position of the arms.

Remember to keep the arm swing straight forwards and backwards instead of across the body. They should not cross the body as this twists the hips, placing more stress on the core muscles and lower back.

Don't clench your hands; relax the fingers in a curled position.

The **stride length of the legs should be increased** and the toes of the front foot need to be pulled up towards the knees as you stride forwards.

This action ensures that your toes don't catch the ground as you walk. The problem with this action is that it can cause a tightness in the muscles down the front of the shins, but *this is something that becomes less of a concern the more often the technique is practiced.*

If you notice a tightening in these muscles, you can do a Tibialis anterior stretch as shown in the section on stretching.

You also need to point your toes out to the sides slightly to aid balance and increase speed.

The heel again needs to take the impact of the stride, but with level 3 walking you should concentrate your thoughts on driving off the back foot to generate more speed and power.

The whole body needs to lean forwards slightly, but from the ankles and not the waist as this places too much stress on the lower back muscles. It's easier to imagine the position of leaning forwards when walking up stairs and try to replicate this in your level 3 walking technique.

Level 4 Walking:

This is the most challenging type of walking there is and it's very demanding. You'll notice that this technique isn't used in the programs until you've developed a good understanding and level of fitness walking technique beforehand.

If you've ever seen walkers at the Olympics on TV, this is the technique they use and they can reach incredibly fast speeds.

For our purposes however, it's an opportunity to use more muscles and increase the calorie expenditure of our sessions. It also adds variety and change to stimulate both body and mind.

Whilst level 4 is a challenging exercise it still has the benefits of being very low impact compared to running and so is an excellent choice for anyone who is overweight or a little older.

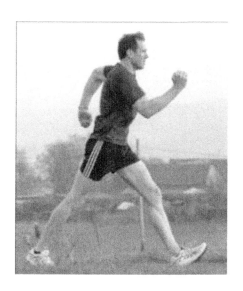 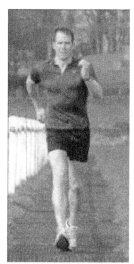 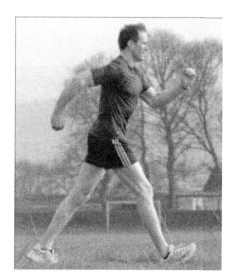

This is how to do it...

Check your posture first, keep your head up, your shoulders back, pull in your tummy muscles and remember the idea of the string running up through your body pulling taut.

Now on to the action itself...

You need to bend your elbows to 90 degrees and fix this position.

The arm movement in level 4 walking should be very pronounced and powerful as it's this that helps to generate more speed and power.

When swinging the arms, it's best not to allow the hands to travel higher than the shoulders on the way forwards because going higher than this doesn't assist in the technique, it can actually hinder it.

The back swing is vital to increasing speed so really get the arms moving.

Remember to keep your elbows fixed at a right angle.

For level 4 walking you need to increase the speed still further and you can do this by speeding up the steps which is easiest done by shortening the stride.

You'll find that because you're walking faster, with slightly shorter strides the pelvis will rotate more, this is natural. You'll also need to narrow your feet position, so that you are not striding out to the sides, instead stepping more inwardly.

The toe lift needs to be increased even more using this technique.

One of the best ways to think of level 4 walking is to **imagine that you are placing one foot in front of the other on an imaginary line as if walking on a tightrope.**

Because you're using this technique your feet will naturally not point out as far to the sides as in level 3.

It's important to lean forwards and again this should come from the heels instead of the lower back.

When practicing level 4 walking try firstly without the tightrope technique and then by using it.

There should be an increase in speed when using the leg movement in level 4, but just be aware, it will take practice to get right.

If at first you find using the arm motion tiring, just use it for short period of time, perhaps 5 or 10 minute intervals. Try and avoid over striding in an attempt to increase your speed. You place yourself at a much greater risk of injury by doing this.

Your stride should be longer behind your body, where your toe is pushing off, rather than out in front of your body.

Remember it's the back leg that generates power, so it's vital that you get the full power from the push of the back leg as it rolls from heel to toe.

The best way of thinking about walking faster is to try and increase the number of steps you take each second instead of trying to increase your stride length as this can actually slow you down.

Stretching

The more you exercise and walk, the more prone you become to muscular imbalances. The lower back, calves and hamstrings can become tight and inflexible while the shins, quadriceps and stomach muscles may actually get weaker in comparison. Stretching will help to counteract this.

Flexibility is one of the most often overlooked parts of our health and fitness. Flexibility naturally reduces with age but also as you start to increase the amount of time you walk for you will notice that your muscles seem to be getting a little tighter.

Always warm the muscles up first before stretching by walking briskly for 5 minutes as this helps to increase heat in the area making the muscles more pliable and less likely to tear if stretched too vigorously. So, this means if you want to stretch off before exercising you should do so after an initial warm up period.

Stretching off before exercise is not necessary, but **the really important time to stretch off is after exercise**. During exercise the muscles contract repeatedly leading to slightly shorter and tighter muscles, which need help to be lengthened and stretched out. This is where stretching is very helpful as it returns the muscles to their pre-exercise length.

Regular stretching offers the following benefits:

- Helps prevent muscular aches, pains and cramping.
- Reduces the possibility of muscular soreness over the following days.
- Decreases the possibility of suffering muscle strain or injuries.
- Increases the muscle's ability to lengthen and stretch during exercise.
- Improves the muscle's ability to work faster, harder and more efficiently.
- Allows you to safely improve stride length.
- **Improves overall posture** and walking technique.

How to stretch:

Stretching involves taking the muscle to the point of its greatest range of motion, without overextending it. Done correctly you should get a slight feeling of tightness or mild discomfort at about 6 or 7 on the RPE scale (see page 43), not a sharp or shooting pain, this would indicate that you are stretching too far and should ease back a little.

This sharp pain is called the stretch reflex and its job is to ensure that you don't take the muscles further in to a stretch than they are comfortably able to go.

The way we improve flexibility is by working with the stretch reflex which is known as developmental stretching. You can do this as follows:

- Get into a stretch position and take the muscle to a point where you can feel a mild discomfort, just a little further back from where you felt a sharper pain (the stretch reflex)
- Wait for approximately 15 – 20 seconds without pushing any further until the discomfort becomes milder and then ease slowly further into the stretch until

you again feel the stretch reflex. Ease back a little from here and hold this position.

- This can be repeated a few times, but ideally you should move on to another muscle after a minute to avoid stressing the muscle too far.

When stretching after walking you need to focus on all the main muscles groups you've used in your session (see page 20 for a diagram showing these muscles). These are:

Quadriceps	Muscles that run down the front of your thighs, crossing the knee and hip joints
Hamstrings	Muscles that run down on the back of the legs
Adductors	Muscles on the inside of the thighs at the top of the legs
Hip Flexors	Muscles at the top and front of the thighs
Gluteus Maximus	Muscles of the buttocks
Gastrocnemus	The longest muscle in the calves just below the knee
Soleus	The shorter muscle of the calves just above the ankle

Make sure you follow these guidelines to avoid injury when stretching:

- Do not overextend the muscles.
- You should feel very minimal tightness/discomfort (but not pain)
- Hold and control the stretch for at least 15 - 30 seconds.
- Stretch all the major leg muscle groups as listed above.
- Stretch uniformly (after stretching one leg, stretch the other)
- **Don't overstretch an injured area as this may cause additional damage.**
- Never bounce when stretching as this can increase your chances of suffering an injury!

Always include stretching after a long or challenging walk, make it part of the training and cool down process, get into the habit.

Your legs will be the most receptive to the benefits of stretching straight after you walk because they'll be warmer and more pliable. Stretch gently and slowly and while your muscles are still warm.

If your flexibility is quite poor, a regular program of stretching will help to rectify the problem, stretching every day is a good idea, but always after you have warmed the muscles up first.

Roadside Stretches

Gastrocnemius (upper calf) Stretch

- Stand tall with one leg in front of the other, hands flat and at shoulder height against a wall

- Keep your hips facing the wall with the rear leg and spine in a straight line and bend your front leg

- Push against the wall and press the back heel into the ground, there shouldn't be any pressure on the front foot

- You should feel the stretch in the calf of the straight leg

- Repeat with the other leg

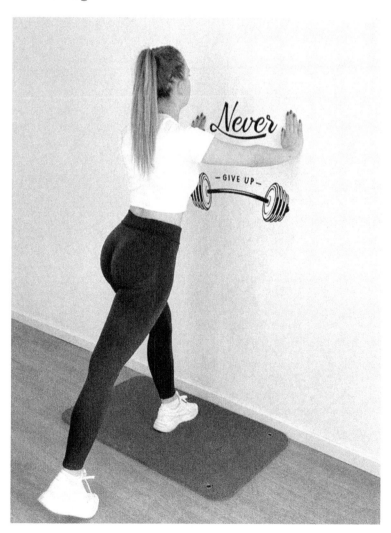

Soleus (lower calf) Stretch

• Standing as above, bring your back foot in closer to the wall and bend the bent leg a little further

• Keep both feet flat on the floor- you should feel a stretch in your lower calf of the back leg

• Leaning towards the wall intensifies the stretch

• There should be little pressure on the front foot

• Repeat with the other leg

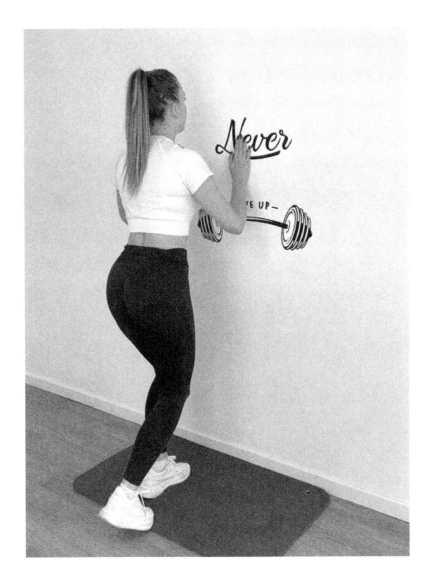

Standing Quadriceps (front of thigh) Stretch

• Lean against a wall and bend your right knee, grasping the right foot with your right hand behind you

• Lift your foot backwards until your heel is as close as possible to the buttocks, without touching

• Flex your foot and keep your body straight

• Push the hips a little further forward if you can't feel the stretch down the front of the thighs

• Repeat with the other leg.

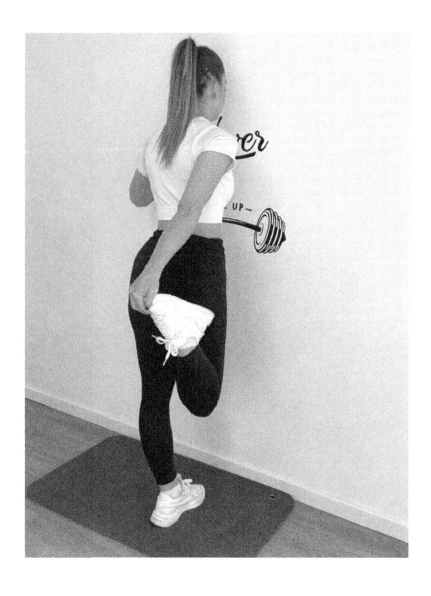

Hamstring (back of thigh) Stretch

• Stand with your left foot placed flat on the ground in front of you and keep your extended leg straight

• Bend the right thigh, stick your bottom out and place your hands on your bent leg for support

• Lean forwards into your straight leg, pushing your bottom out, then straighten your upper body until you can feel a stretch down the back of the straight leg

• Repeat with the other leg

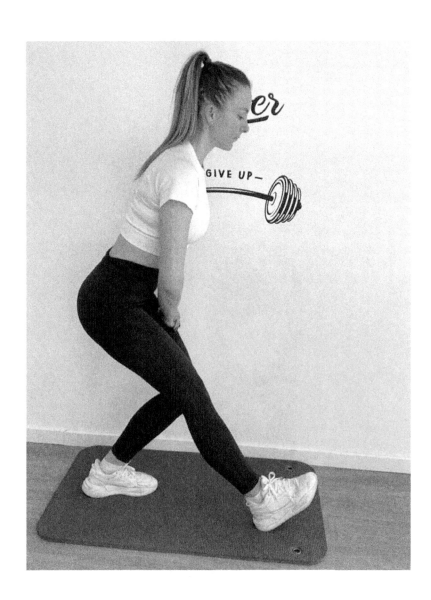

Hip Flexor (front of upper thigh) Stretch

• Take a long lunge forward

• Keep your hips square and your upper body vertical

• Place your hands on your front thigh

• Dip your back knee towards the ground until you feel a stretch down the back thigh, high up towards the top of your leg

• Repeat with the other leg

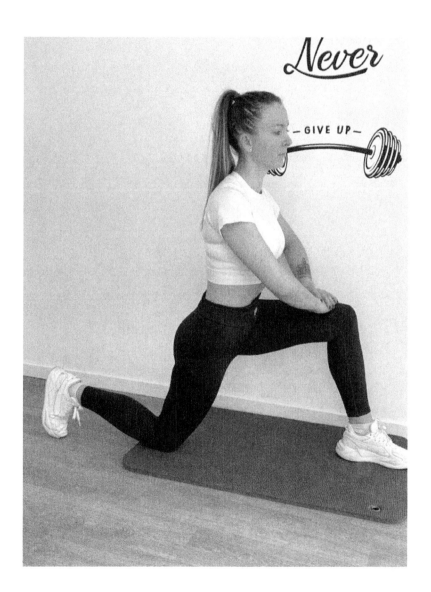

Adductor (inner thigh) Stretch

- Stand tall with both feet pointing forwards, approximately two shoulders width apart

- Bend the right leg, place both hands on the bent thigh and lower the body towards the ground, keeping the left leg straight

- Keep your back straight and chest out

- You should feel this stretch high up the leg on the inside just below the groin of the straight leg

- Repeat with the other leg

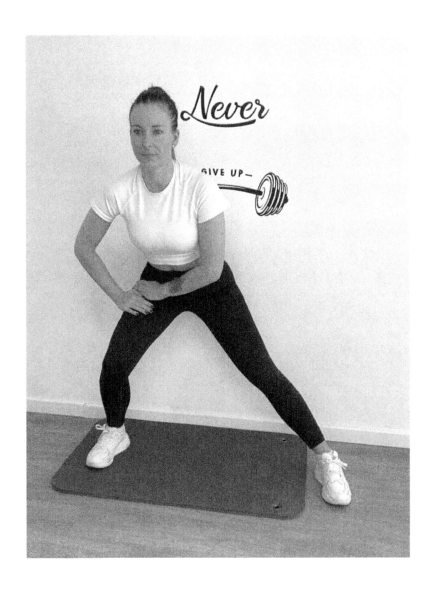

Standing Glute (buttocks) Stretch

- Lean with your back against a wall for support

- Take hold of your right leg with both arms around the calf

- Pull in towards the chest until you can feel a stretch down the back of the right buttock

- Repeat with the other leg

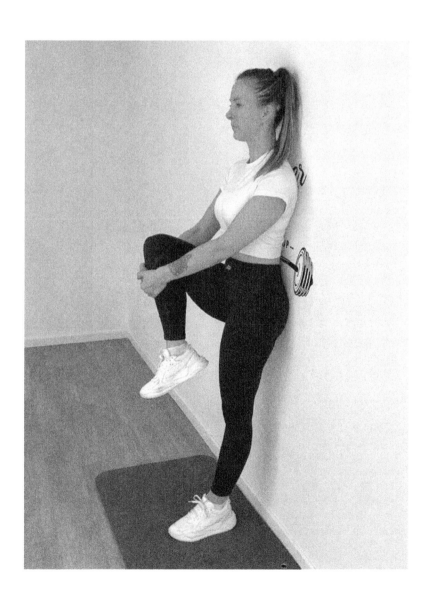

Standing Tibialis Stretch

• Stand with your feet a hips width apart and your knees slightly bent

• Bend your right knee and grasp the toes of your right foot with your right hand, move your right knee forward

• Pull up on your toes forcing the top of your foot towards the ground

• You should feel this stretch down the front of the right shin

• Place one hand against a wall for balance if necessary

• Repeat with the other leg

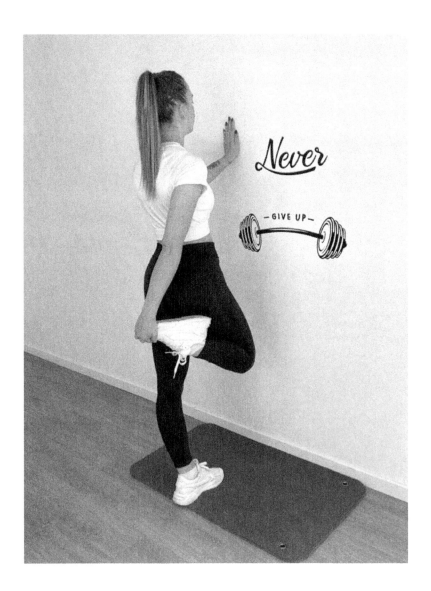

Combined Stretches

The stretching techniques below allow you to stretch a number of muscles at the same time, which means you can stretch much quicker. These can be done at home where you can use either a mat or towel to sit on.

Lying Quadriceps and Tibialis Stretch

● Sit down on to the floor on your bent knees with your buttocks on top of your feet

● Make sure the tops of your feet are flat on the floor with your toes pointing towards your back

● Gently lean backwards as far as you can comfortably go until you can feel the stretch down the front of the thighs and the shins

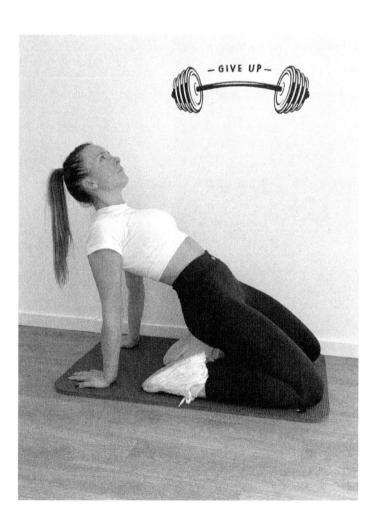

Hamstring and Adductor Stretch

• Sit on the ground with both legs straight out in front of you

• Bend the left leg and place the sole of the left foot alongside the knee of the right leg

• Allow the right leg to lie relaxed on the ground and bend forward, keeping the back straight

• You should feel the stretch down the back of the left leg and inside of the right upper thigh

• Repeat with the other leg

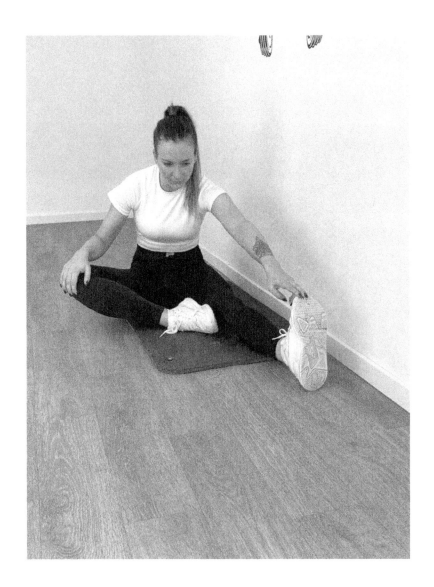

Simultaneous Gastrocnemius Stretch

• Using a wall for support, place both hands against it and take a wide stride backwards

• Keep both heels flat on the floor

• Lean forwards keeping your back and legs straight

• You should feel this stretch in both calves at the same time

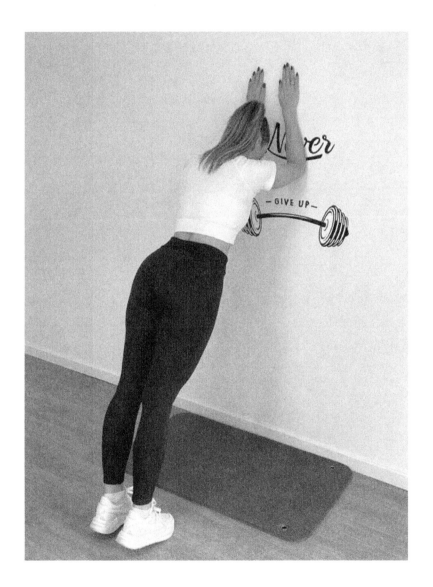

Gluteus and Lower Back Stretch

- Lying on the floor on your back

- Wrap both arms around the front of the shins and pull the thighs in towards the body

- Round your spine and hold that position

- You should be feeling this stretch on the lower back and around the buttocks

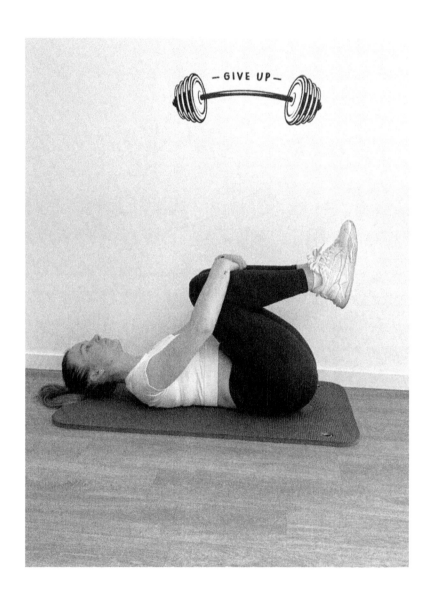

Final Thoughts

DON'T STRETCH COLD MUSCLES.

It's far better to stretch after a walk than before one.

Do stretch lightly before doing any challenging workouts (after a short 5 minute warm up) and during any exercise sessions where you feel your muscles tightening up halfway through.

Ease into your stretches gently, *don't bounce or force them*.

After a walk, hold each stretch for 30 seconds and repeat once or twice on each leg.

Equipment

Walking Gadgets

As time progresses, the technology we have at our fingertips also improves and over the last few years there have been some very important developments in the area of tracking and monitoring how far and how fast you walk.

Pedometer

The humble pedometer now seems like a very basic type of instrument, but it can still provide some useful information.

A pedometer or step counter is a portable device that counts each step a person takes by detecting the movement of their hips. Because the distance of each person's step varies, you'll need to adjust it before using it.

Pedometers are usually worn on a belt or waistband and used to record how many steps the wearer has walked or run, and then it calculates the distance walked in either kilometres or miles based on the stride length that's been programmed in by the user.

Step counters are also being integrated into an increasing number of portable electronic devices such as mp3 players and mobile phones, which use shoe sensors that transmit information to a wireless receiver.

Workout information such as elapsed time, distance travelled, and calories burned can all be recorded.

Unfortunately, some basic pedometers accidentally record movements other than walking, such as bending over to tie a shoelace, or bumps from the road when travelling in a car or bus etc, but the more advanced and expensive versions record fewer of these 'false steps'.

Another criticism of the standard pedometer is that it can't record intensity, but you can work around this by setting step targets within a certain time limit, e.g. 1000 steps in a certain amount of time.

Heart Rate Monitor

A heart rate monitor allows you to measure and record your heart rate. These usually consist of two parts, a chest transmitter attached by an adjustable fabric strap and a wrist receiver, mobile phone or other device.

Advanced versions can also measure variances in your heart rate and breathing rate to assess and monitor your level of fitness. When a heartbeat is detected, a radio or digital signal is transmitted, which the receiver picks up to record the current heart rate.

Heart rate monitors may give you some or all of the following information:

- Average heart rate over exercise period.
- Time spent working in a specific heart rate zone.
- Calories burned over the course of the walk.
- Breathing rate.
- Distance covered (using GPS tracking)
- Average speed (using GPS tracking)

This information can often be downloaded to a computer, depending on which version of heart rate monitor you buy.

Stopwatch

A stopwatch is a handheld timer designed to measure the amount of time elapsed from a particular point when started to when the timer is stopped.

Typically, the timing functions are controlled by two buttons on the casing. Pressing one button starts the timer, and pressing the button a second time stops it, leaving the elapsed time displayed. A press of another button then resets the stopwatch to zero.

The second button can often be used to record split times or lap times. When the split time button is pressed while the timer is running, the display freezes, allowing the elapsed time to that point to be read, but the timer mechanism continues to record the total time. Pressing the split button a second time allows the watch to resume display of total time elapsed. This could be useful if you're doing a route a number of times, to measure the average time taken per lap.

Many wrist watches, mobile phones and music players have a stopwatch function, so it's worth checking to see if you have any of these before committing to buying one.

GPS Walking Technology

Global Positioning System (GPS) is a satellite system developed by the United States Department of Defence for their own air force. It can be used by individuals to track journeys and distances both on and off road all over the world.

The system relies on using between 24 and 32 satellites to transmit precise radio wave signals, which allow GPS receivers to determine their current location, time and speed.

GPS systems adapted for walking or running are excellent tools for calculating and tracking your own training and progress. However, before you choose a GPS watch, phone, or other device, it is important to understand how it can be used to improve your training.

One method is simply to use your GPS to record the distance you've walked if you've decided on a target, for example 3 miles.

Position tracking (for tracking your location) can also be very helpful if you are doing long distances, so you don't get lost, particularly if you're in a more rural location.

GPS is also useful in tracking speed-based goals. Rather than just tracking the distance you are walking; you can focus on the pace at which you are travelling these distances at.

With any good GPS system, you can normally expect accuracy to be within a few feet. However, the satellite signals are not able to pass through structures, so if you are out of the direct view of a satellite you probably won't get an accurate signal, or one possibly reflected off another structure nearby. In this case the signal will have travelled further and so your calculated position could be_incorrect. This is called 'a multipath error'. It's a very common problem in built up areas such as in towns and cities.

Areas that have a poor reception, overhead trees, foliage and weather conditions such as clouds, rain, snow etc can also have an impact on the signals you receive. These conditions can weaken signals to the point where they are unusable.

Generally speaking, you can expect newer models to be more reliable and sensitive than the older ones.

Running Watch

A running watch is a very handy training aid to have. The good news is that most are surprisingly easy to use, with prompts on screen telling you which mode you have entered and what happens if you hold down a particular key etc.

There are some basic requirements you will need to consider before making a purchase such as whether the screen is readable at arm's length? Are the buttons easy to use whilst walking?

You'll find that a specialist running watch is far more than just a time device, but also offers users a variety of training options and it may even include GPS tracking.

Some of the more advanced watches have even more features, such as heart rate monitors and calorie counters as well as some of the following features:

- Countdown timer: Some watches also have countdown timers. This can be helpful if you're doing repetitions or you're on a warm-down and want to have a countdown rather than up.

- Stopwatch Mode: The stopwatch mode times your walks in hours, minutes, seconds and fractions of a second.

- Memory: Some watches can keep a record of your lap times and splits (different periods of time or distance) for example your 1-mile splits. When you enter the memory recall mode, each workout has a page showing the date and overall time of the session.

- You are then able to select which session you want to view and then scroll through lap by lap or split by split. Some watches can also highlight the session's best lap and calculate your average lap time. Once you've finished viewing, you can choose whether to delete the session from the memory or keep it for future reference.

All these gadgets are simply tools that allow you to get more information about how you are progressing, which is a very important factor.

When you are training hard and regularly, it is important to know exactly how far you have come and how far you still have to go.

My advice is to buy a good heart rate monitor which also includes GPS tracking features. This way you have access to all the information you need. Your heart rates, distances, speeds and times.

Mobile Phone

I would always advise any walker to carry a mobile phone for your own health, safety and wellbeing.

You may witness an accident or be involved in one yourself, get lost or suffer an injury which means you need help getting home.

IT'S ALWAYS USEFUL TO HAVE A WAY OF CONTACTING SOMEONE WHEN YOU ARE OUT WALKING, JUST IN CASE.

Equipment List:

For the most part you won't need a lot of equipment to head out walking, but my essential list would be:

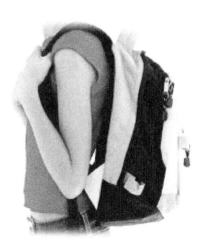

- Mobile phone (in case of emergencies)
- Timer / Watch.
- Spare money for a bus or taxi (in case you need to get home quickly)
- Water bottle – to keep you hydrated.

However, if you're planning a longer trip, or are going to walk off-road, you might need other things with you.

Here's a quick list of some other things you may or may not need to take with depending on the type of walking you're doing…

- A lightweight rucksack to hold your equipment (wear both shoulder straps to make sure the weight is evenly distributed around your back, or you could strain one side of your back)
- Some sunscreen if it's hot and sunny.
- Waterproofs and a hat if it's cold and wet.
- A map if you're walking long distances and are unsure of the area you're walking in.
- Walking poles if you're going off the beaten track and walking on uneven ground. These can be a great help to balance you when you're going up or down any particularly challenging hills or mountains.
- A whistle and luminous clothing if you are going hill walking in remote areas.
- A sugary snack, cereal bar, or piece of fruit if you're going on a very long walk and you feel your blood sugar levels dropping.
- **A first aid kit.**
- A lightweight fleece jumper (if it turns cold)

Safety

Essential Safety Tips

Once you've committed to your walking plan, you'll be spending quite a bit of your time walking outdoors and inevitably some of this walking will take place on or near roads. Your safety should be your priority.

Here are some tips and ideas to keep you safe.

When you're crossing roads, the best way to avoid accidents is to be prepared and be aware of vehicles around you. Here are some safety tips to follow:

Walk on pavements: If pavements aren't available, walk on the edge of the road or on the shoulder, facing the traffic flow. Use pedestrian bridges when they are available.

Use marked crossing points: Pedestrians are most often hit by cars when they cross the road where there are no crossing points.

TAKE YOUR TIME AND CROSS SAFELY

Look left, right, and left for traffic: Stop at the curb and look left, right, and left again for traffic. Stopping at the curb signals to drivers that you intend to cross. Always obey traffic signals.

See and be seen: Drivers need to see you to avoid you.

- Stay out of the driver's blind spot.

- Make eye contact with drivers when crossing busy streets.
- Wear bright colours or reflective clothing if you are walking near traffic at night.
- **Carry a flashlight when walking in the dark.**
- In bad weather, take care that your umbrella or raincoat doesn't stop drivers from seeing you.

Drinking and walking? Alcohol can impair the judgment and motor skills of pedestrians just as it does for drivers. Don't take unnecessary risks by drinking before walking, just as you wouldn't with driving. Take the bus, take a cab, or have a friend drive you home.

Beware of the effects of prescription and non-prescription medications and drugs too.

Obey traffic signals: At crossing points pedestrians must obey the signals and not cross against the stop signal unless specifically directed to go by a traffic officer.

No matter where you choose to do your walking for weight loss workouts, you must always consider the safety aspects of the places you choose to walk.

Safety When Walking Alone

Women need to take extra care when walking alone, and there are a number of things that will help you to stay safe:

1. Plan a few different routes so that you avoid walking the same route at predictable times.

2. Make sure someone reliable knows your route and an expected time of return.

3. Walk in busy, well-lit, familiar areas and steer clear of parks and riverbanks. **If you have a mobile phone, take it with you.**

Make sure you're aware of what's going on around you, listening to music decreases your awareness particularly of what's behind you. You may want to consider any of the personal alarms on the market that are small enough to carry when walking and perhaps a whistle as well. If you get in trouble a whistle will draw attention and would probably get you help faster than anything else.

If you see anything unusual or suspicious report it to the police. Make eye contact with people you pass - looking away indicates fear. Make a mental note of the places along your route where you can find help. Walk with your dog if you have one, attackers are often deterred by dogs, even small ones.

If you feel you are being followed, or are attacked, draw attention to yourself. Attackers don't want to be noticed or identified. If you cause a commotion, they are more likely to leave you alone.

You are more likely to escape if you fight back. Kick, scream and gouge (eyes, windpipe and groin are all good targets). Keys, pepper spray, or even a pen can be used as a weapon. To get help quickly in case of being attacked shout 'FIRE', this is more likely to get people to come to your aid than just shouting 'HELP'

If you walk alone, carry self-defence/pepper spray, but make sure you know how to use it and that it is legal in your country. During an attack is no time to realize you don't know how it works. Some sprays come with a convenient practice canister. In the case of a dog attack, pepper spray might not always work. In the unlikely event you are subject to a dog attack stop moving, dogs like a moving target, curl up in foetal position, and protect head and neck. If you drive to your favorite walking location, don't leave valuables in plain sight in the car. It's an open invitation for theft.

Another good option is to join a walking club. You can walk with them and keep safe, but more importantly you will make friends with other walkers in your local area and you may then be able to arrange regular companions for walks – there's safety in numbers.

Don't be paranoid about walking on your own as it's very rare that anything bad will happen, but it's important that you are aware of the potential risks and take reasonable precautions against anything happening to you.

Walking at Night

It makes more sense to walk during the day, but walking at night may be your only option if its winter or if you have a hectic diary juggling work, family and your social life.

However, walking in the dark means a certain amount of risk.

On the one hand you should try to walk where there are other people around and in well-lit areas, but on the other hand, the extra traffic in these places may mean risks from fast moving traffic.

Here are some safety tips to follow to ensure that you make it through your night time walks without incident or accident.

Always Walk Facing Oncoming Traffic: When walking in the dark, you should **always walk on the side of the road that faces oncoming traffic**. This allows you to see vehicles approaching you, making it far easier and safer to keep away from them.

Walking in the dark is always much harder because of the poor visibility levels due to the glare of headlamps and overhead street lighting. Because of this you should only select routes that have pavements or purpose-built walkways. Don't use very busy roads to walk on at night.

Be Safe, Be Seen: Ideally you should wear lighter colour clothing. White, yellow or orange clothing tends to be seen much easier in the dark. Luminous or reflective materials are even better. These are widely available in specialist walking or running shops and you can often find arm bands, reflective hats, badges, or sashes that will all make you more visible.

Take a mobile with you: **All walkers should carry a mobile phone with them** regardless of the time of day they walk at. You may pick up an injury and be unable to continue, you may get lost or too tired to carry on or witness an accident or crime etc. These are all very good reasons for carrying a phone with you.

Another good suggestion is to always carry identification. A driver's license will do. You can keep this easily in your pocket or in a hip bag.

Walk with Others: You can walk on your own at any time, but often it can be very motivating and safer to walk with others, either as part of a walking or rambling club or with a friend. Alternatively, why not go walking with a dog, your own or one borrowed from a friend. The dog will love it and you may be saving your friend or neighbour having to go out to walk it!

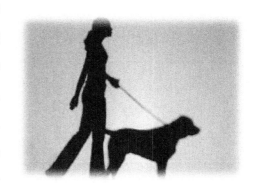

Walking at night can be a wonderful experience, it's a great chance to unwind after a hard day at work, or it can give you chance to get away from the family for an hour or so.

Whatever the reason, take reasonable precautions for your own safety.

Walking in the Rain

Walking in the rain can be an invigorating experience, one where you feel you're beating the elements and mastering your own fitness at the same time.

The sensation of a hot shower after being soaked by the rain is a very uplifting and rewarding end to a great workout.

There are a few extra factors you need to consider when walking in the rain. Here are my top 5 golden rules for walking in the rain...

1. Wear layers	Wear layers of clothes rather than just one top. Waterproof jackets can actually irritate the skin after a while, so ideally you should wear a lightweight vest or T-shirt underneath it, preferably a sweat wicking fabric as waterproof jackets can make you sweat more than usual.
2. Wear waterproofs	Wear a windproof, waterproof jacket whenever you plan to go walking in the rain, but beware of using cheaper jackets as they will not only keep water out, but also hold the moisture from within, leaving you feel clammy and cold.
3. Wear a hat	Wear a hat with a brim or peak so the rain doesn't run in your eyes. Rain on your face can be very uncomfortable. Also, if the area you walk in is particularly built up the rain could be polluted and quite acidic, which could irritate your eyes if the water gets in them.
4. Wear bright clothing	**Make sure you wear bright and ideally reflective clothing**. When you're walking in the rain not only will you find it difficult to see far in front of you, but other road users will too, especially in heavy rainfall. So, m*ake sure you're easy to spot on a rainy day.*
5. Don't overdress	It might be raining, but that doesn't mean it's cold out. If you wear too many thick layers without a waterproof jacket, your clothing will become wet, uncomfortable and heavy. Dress correctly for the weather.

One last point to mention when you've been walking in the rain is to take care of your training shoes by filling them up with old newspaper or kitchen towelling rolled into balls after you've arrived back home. This keeps your shoes in good shape by drawing the moisture away from the fabric and insole.

What's Next

Advanced Training Techniques

Once you've got your walking program up and running and you're getting into the swing of things, you'll need to try something new and perhaps a bit more challenging. The next few pages will take you through some of the advanced walking techniques you'll find in the programs.

Using these advanced techniques will help to...

- Keep your training interesting, enjoyable and challenging.
- Ensure that your mind and body is given regular stimulation for change.
- Dramatically boost fitness and fat loss levels far quicker than simply walking at the same pace and in similar circumstances each session.

These training techniques can feel quite hard at first, but **it's absolutely vital to push yourself a little further on a regular basis** in order to improve your ability to do more in the future, in fact it's the only way you will ever improve.

If you don't add new things into your routine, you could start to stagnate and never increase your mileage or endurance.

It's great that you've got started but you need to continue to push yourself.

Building up your endurance by gradually increasing the distances you walk is just one way of improving your fitness and losing weight. To continue to make progress as quickly as possible and burn more calories you can use a selection of the following advanced walking techniques.

Hills

If you are lucky enough (or unlucky – depending on your viewpoint) to live near hills, you can start to use these in your training. Hill training offers a great way to add intensity and build up power and strength in the legs.

Adding hill reps to your walking program adds a much-needed dimension to a longer walk, allowing muscle groups to function at anaerobic levels for a short period of time.   In addition, hills and off-road walking strengthen the muscles and connective tissues surrounding the ankles which are an area of the body that is subjected to the most stress when walking because the ankles provide balance and stability to the whole body.

Obviously if you live in an area where there aren't any hills you can't do this outside, but you can use a treadmill either at home or at your local gym. **Using a treadmill for some of your walking is actually a good idea** because of the reduced impact on your joints due to the cushioned effect of the treadmill walking belt and bed.

Walking hills can help in the following ways:

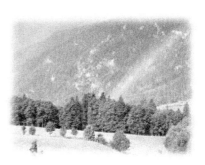

- Develops control and stabilization in your body and joints (downhill walking)
- Promotes strength and endurance in the legs (uphill walking)
- Helps to develop maximum speed and power.
- Improves the body's ability to handle lactic acid.

How to get started: In order to do hill reps, you should select a hill or a section of a hill that will take you approximately 1 – 2 minutes to walk up, the steeper the better.

You'll be walking up this at a steady pace, so don't go too far to begin with.

Walk up hill using the recommended speed as shown in the programs and then simply walk back down very gently so as to protect your joints. Before you start your hill reps, you'll need to warm up properly, brisk walking on a flat level and then stretching should be fine.

Remember to also cool down at the end, again followed by stretches. The rest of the time should be work/rest time. Rest between hill reps should be as long as it takes for you to reach a comfortable 5/6 on the RPE scale and your breathing rate has lowered considerably. If this takes 5 minutes or just 30 seconds, wait until you have recovered.

Make a note on your training log of the length of time you walk each rep, how long you rest for, and how many reps you manage to do in the allotted workout time.

Interval Training

Using interval training in your workouts is a great way to increase your fitness and **burn more calories because it allows you to take periods of relative rest after periods of higher intensity exercise.** This helps your body to clear lactic acid away from the working muscles leaving your legs ready to continue further.

With intervals there are many ways you can organise the session and it really is up to you. The main point to remember is that there should be a definite structure to the session which should be decided beforehand.

One common interval training approach is to begin with a rest/work ratio of 4:1 (e.g. slow walking or rest for 4 minutes, work for 1 minute), then the following week as your fitness improves 3:1, then 2:1 and so on. Use this basis if you like, or the suggestions in the program breakdowns or change to suit your preferences.

Also, you're not limited to intervals of hard and easy walking, you could try something like the following program…

Level 1 pace for 1 minute, level 2 pace for 1 minute and then walk at level 3 pace for 30 seconds.

It really is up to you. Make sure you record the details of your workout in your training log and subsequent sessions are increased by either the time as I have shown or the level of intensity you use.

One technique to use is to walk slowly to one lamp post, then quickly to the next, then slowly again and so on. Both the distance and speed can be changed to add variety to your workouts.

Using interval training in your program means that you can often reduce the amount of training but still continue to see improvements in your fitness levels and walking performance.

The recovery interval could consist of simply strolling at level 1 walking pace in order to bring down your heart rate, ideally to an RPE of approximately 5-6 out of 10 by the end of the recovery bout. As you get fitter, your heart rate will drop much faster, allowing you to recover more efficiently.

The benefits of interval training:

- Very efficient and effective method of burning fat and boosting your metabolic rate.
- Improves maximum oxygen uptake and increases fitness levels.
- Interval training is a more challenging and more interesting way of training compared to walking at the same pace for longer distances.

Fartlek Training

Fartlek training means 'playing with speed'. It is an advanced training technique which relies on your own judgement and level of fatigue. **It's a great way to move your training forwards**, without the structure of interval training.

The idea behind Fartlek training is to walk all of the session, but intersperse that with periods of faster walking, as and when you feel capable of doing so.

Fartlek is a Swedish word meaning "speed play." The use of 'Fartlek' came about to provide a less structured approach to that of interval training. The benefits of this type of training are that it allows you to *increase or lower the intensity* of your training **depending on how you're feeling.**

Fartlek training is generally used to improve aerobic fitness and your ability to cope with higher levels of lactic acid build up in the muscles. It combines fast and slow walking within a continuous walk. Stages of faster walking are followed by easy recovery walking. The length of speed bursts and recovery should be unstructured so that you can get a real feeling of playing with speed.

Since the aim of Fartlek training is to develop speed, the general pace should be relatively easy, although the overall effect of this type of training is far from easy.

Only the speed bursts should be done with any intensity and these short bursts of speed should only be around 30 seconds to one minute to begin with and increasing as you become fitter, although you won't be timing this, instead you'll be gauging how it feels and slowing down when you feel you need to.

Remember, you must leave yourself enough time between each higher paced burst so that you can fully recover in between.

Cross Training

Cross training is simply the use of different types of aerobic exercise in addition to walking to improve your aerobic ability. Anything that challenges your heart a little to improve fitness levels and the strength and endurance of the heart and lungs can contribute to cross training.

Using a wide range of activities to improve fitness levels keeps workouts fresh and enjoyable. This variety also removes much of the stress to the same muscles and joints you will find when continually performing the same type of exercise.

Single sports programmes can often lead to muscle imbalances and repetitive motion injuries. With cross training there is much less likelihood that these injuries will occur due to the variety and range of different muscle groups involved.

Aim to get out of your comfort zone and push yourself towards new highs. Don't be content to simply go through the motions with your cross training, it's ok to do that sometimes, but to get the most benefit, you'll need to progress in some way each workout.

Cross training can include rowing, swimming, cycling, aerobics classes, dance classes, etc. If you choose to do this at a gym, you can use any number of pieces of equipment in one session or just stay on one, it's up to you. Your aim should still be to improve the strength and endurance of your cardiovascular system (heart, lungs and circulation).

Building up the number of times you exercise will also increase your endurance, helping you to increase your distances when you go walking. All of the walking programs contain cross training at some point or another.

Pyramid Training

Pyramid training is a way of gradually increasing the intensity you are working at. You begin at a gentle pace and gradually increase the speed to a peak in the middle. Then you gradually slow the pace back down to the end of the session. The secret here is to work very hard in the middle for a short period of time only, building up from the beginning and tapering down towards the end.

If you plan on using a heart rate monitor for this exercise, you'll need to work out your heart rates for each increase. Work out 50-60%, 60 -70%, 70 – 80% and 80 – 90% of your maximum heart rate.

You can use this formula: 220 – Your age = maximum heart rate.

(E.g. a man who is 50 years old has a maximum heart rate of 170)

So, to work out 50 % of his maximum heart rate you can simply divide 170 ÷ 10 and then times this by 5. 17 x 5 = 85

If our 50 year-old man wants to work at 50% of his maximum heart rate he would need to keep his heart rate at or around 85 beats per minute (Bpm).

To start pyramid training, you should warm up gently for about 5 minutes and then start your training spending 2 – 5 minutes in each heart rate or RPE zone building up to a peak at RPE 9/10 or

80 – 90% of your maximum heart rate in the middle of your session and then working back down again, finishing with a cool down and stretch of all the major muscles worked.

A typical 24 minute pyramid workout for our example 50 year-old male would look something like this:

220 – 50 = 170 maximum heart rate

% Max Heart Rate	Your Heart Rates (Bpm)/RPE Scale (Example 50 year old)		Time
5 minute warm up			
50 - 60%	85 – 102 Bpm /	6	2 minutes
60 - 70%	102 – 119 Bpm /	7	2 minutes
70 - 80%	119 – 136 Bpm /	8	2 minutes
80 - 90%	136 – 153 Bpm /	9	1 - 2 minutes
70 - 80%	119 – 136 Bpm /	8	2 minutes
60 - 70%	102 – 119 Bpm /	7	2 minutes
50 - 60%	85 – 102 Bpm /	6	2 minutes
5 minute cool down			

Using Extra Weight to Increase Intensity

There is a lot of debate about the safety of using extra weight to increase the intensity of workouts.

The main problem with adding weights to your arms or legs is that **it can change the mechanics of the way your body stands and moves**. This can put stress on the supporting and stabilizing muscles, tendons and ligaments which could result in injury.

Adding extra weight is a good way to vary your sessions and make them more challenging, but the best options are to use very light hand weights which have a strap attached to slide your hands through. The weight shouldn't be heavier than 1kg on each hand.

Alternatively, you can buy purpose made water bottles which are designed to fit your grip. You should use one on each hand filled equally for balance.

However, **the safest and most effective thing to use is a weighted vest or belt**. The reason this is a much better option is that weight is distributed on your torso which is the centre of gravity and the way your limbs move will be completely unaffected.

I don't recommend using ankle weights as this will completely change your walking gait.

Treadmill Walking

Using a treadmill can be a great way to maintain your walking schedule if you can't walk outside if the weather is really bad, or if you prefer using the gym.

One important thing about using the gym is that you should keep each session a little varied and progressive, you should do more than the last time you did the same session.

Every session should start with a warm up, 5 minutes of slow to moderately paced walking is enough, the aim is to raise the temperature of the muscles a little and increase the work rate of the heart and warm up the lungs.

Always finish off each workout with a 5 minute cool down, again gentle walking is ideal, followed by the stretches as outlined on pages 38 - 43.

There are many benefits to using a treadmill for your walking sessions. Here are just a few:

- You're at no risk from other road users.
- You can keep warm, dry, cool and out of the sun etc.
- You can accurately record the speed and lengths of time you walk for.
- You'll have no excuses not to go, it'll never be too wet, windy or hot etc.
- The treadmill will never be icy or slippery.
- You can focus purely on your walking.

Perhaps one of the best benefits to using a treadmill is **the control you have over your sessions**. You can increase speed and incline at the press of a button.

This absolute control makes it very easy to progress your sessions as you'll have an accurate measure of exactly what, when and how long you managed to do.

Most treadmills now have heart rate sensors as well so this is another measure you can add to your training log.

Every workout in this manual can be done on a treadmill if you prefer not to do your walking outside.

Off-Road Walking

Walking on different surfaces can add a new challenge as well as some interest to your workouts, but primarily you should walk on whatever surface you feel comfortable on, whether that be grass, sand, road or rugged terrain.

A certain amount of walking should be done on different surfaces, to allow for adaptations in your balance and stabilising and supporting muscles and tendons etc.

Just walking many miles on roads can be a bit tedious as well as lacking the challenge of walking on rugged or uneven terrain.

Walking on differing types of terrain can also help you develop overall strength as this works slightly different muscles. You'll also see more of the world and won't be permanently breathing in the fumes from cars and other vehicles.

How to Start Your Own Walking Club

If you hate the thought of walking on your own **why not start your own walking club**?

Here are some tips for how to start your own walking group.

Get the word around: First of all, you need to *put the word out with the people you know.* Friends, family or work colleagues all provide an excellent network of potential walking group members.

Hopefully from this list you may get a few people interested in joining to start your group off.

From this initial interest, you need to decide which days and times you'll meet. One of the most frustrating things you'll find about organising anything is that *you can't please everyone, and I'd expect that some people may not turn up* if I were you.

It's simpler to stick to just one day a week for a club, eventually if you have enough interest and your club grows in size, then you can walk on more days of the week. Once you have your set time and day organised you can move on to getting more walkers.

Go viral: Join Face book or use your Face book account and send out a message to all your contacts. Make it viral - ask all your contacts to pass the message on to their own contacts.

Not everyone will do this, but if only a few do, you'll have literally hundreds of messages flying around about your new walking club.

Your invitations should include the following details: -

- Who's invited? Is it a mixed gender walking club? Are dogs welcome?
- **Where you'll meet up.**
- How far you'll walk.
- The standard of walking, will it be power walking or just rambling along.
- The time and dates.

Send out emails: You can also send out an email to your walking contact list and again ask all the recipients to forward it on to their contacts.

Use your contacts: Another good place to put the word out about your walking club is your workplace, your partner's workplace, children's school, playgroup or nursery etc.

Put up posters: If you live in a small village or town, put up posters in the shops or libraries etc.

Don't be put off by an initial lack of interest, once you've been going for a while, you'll find that the word will spread.

ONCE YOU BEGIN, YOU'LL NEED TO BE THERE LEADING YOUR WALKS EVERY WEEK, COME RAIN OR SHINE, because the consistency and word of mouth will attract new walkers and so your club will grow.

Nordic Walking

Nordic walking is a technique from Scandinavia, it uses walking poles to increase the amount of effort used.

Originally called ski walking, it uses 2 poles which are similar to those used when skiing. The use of these poles makes it an excellent upper body workout because it challenges the muscles of the upper body at the same time as working the legs.

There is also the added benefit of increased balance and stability that you'll get from using 2 walking poles. Nordic walking is growing in popularity throughout the world and estimates suggest that over 10 million people regularly use this technique to help them stay fit.

It's a great way to exercise outdoors that **doesn't require huge amounts of co-ordination or skill**, although there is a definite technique to using the poles which needs to be learnt to get the most benefit.

It's increasingly being used by fitness professionals and health clubs as another unique and diverse way to improve fitness levels and increase the weight loss of their clients.

It can also be a very social activity. The fact that many classes tend to be set in rural areas also adds to the enjoyment and pleasure of the activity.

Here's a quick summary of some of its biggest benefits:

- It speeds up weight loss, burning up to 20 – 30% more calories than normal strolling.
- Increases the strength of your heart.
- Strengthens most of the muscles of your upper body.
- Reduces the stress on the joints.
- The poles help improve balance and stability.
- Strengthens the bones of the lower and upper body and **can combat the effects of osteoporosis**.
- Reduces the impact of the heels as they strike the ground by up to 30%.

Whilst Nordic walking may well be a great addition to anyone's healthy lifestyle, there are a couple of downsides, firstly the cost of buying good quality walking poles isn't cheap.

You may also feel a little more conspicuous walking along the street using walking poles. This is a drawback to anyone who is a little overweight and uncomfortable about exercising in public as attention will definitely be drawn to you as you walk along.

I **would definitely recommend Nordic walking** as long you aren't concerned about the cost of buying the poles or the funny looks you might get from passers-by. If you don't think it's for you then don't worry because you can easily get similar benefits by using your arms in the power walking techniques found in this walking guide.

The Exercise Schedules

Schedule 1 – Absolute Beginners (suitable for unfit or injured people)

This schedule is meant for anyone who is recovering from any injuries, illness or currently very overweight or particularly unfit. **This is not a typical beginners walking schedule** and is designed to get the user up to comfortably starting the beginners walking schedule 2.

You'll notice that all the sessions use level 1 walking for the first 4 weeks and I have broken sessions down in to very short and manageable chunks, for example 2 x 5 minutes (two walks done separately throughout the day for 5 minutes each).

The duration and intensity of sessions increases along with fitness levels throughout the course of the 6 weeks. You'll be walking most days to begin with on this program unless you feel particularly unwell or tired on the odd occasion.

- When performing any hills sessions, you should actually be walking uphill for the stated time, so for example if the schedule lists '5 minutes hills' I want you to walk up hill for the full 5 minutes.

   This is easily done if you're using a treadmill, but if you're relying on walking up hills, then you may need to go up and down the same one a few times. Don't rush the downhill part as this is not the aim of the session. Unless otherwise written you should walk uphill using level 1 walking speed.

- On any interval sessions throughout Schedule 1, you should use both level 1 and level 2 and structure it this way - walk at level 1 for 1 minute and then level 2 for 1 minute and then repeat for the allotted amount of time.
- You'll notice that a rest or cross training day is added in week 4 as the intensity of the sessions increases. This simply means doing nothing or if you feel fine and want to be active then do 30 minutes of an activity other than walking.

Remember to stretch of thoroughly after each session.

If you want to progress from Schedule 1 on to Schedule 2, then I recommend that you complete all of schedule 1 first and then move on to schedule 2, but start from week 3, not from the beginning.

Schedule 1 – Walking 4 Weight Loss, Very Unfit Beginners Program

WEEKS	MONDAY	TUESDAY	WEDNESDAY	THURSDAY	FRIDAY	SATURDAY	SUNDAY
1	5 Minutes x 2 Level 1	5 Minutes x 2 Level 1	5 Minutes x 2 Level 1	5 Minutes x 2 Level 1	10 Minutes Level 1	10 Minutes Level 1	15 Minutes Level 1
2	8 Minutes x 2 Level 1	8 Minutes x 2 Level 1	8 Minutes x 2 Level 1	10 Minutes Level 1	12 Minutes Level 1	15 Minutes Level 1	20 Minutes Level 1
3	10 Minutes x 2 Level 1	10 Minutes x 2 Level 1	10 Minutes x 2 Level 1	15 Minutes Level 1	5 Minutes Hills	20 Minutes Level 1	25 Minutes Level 1
4	15 Minutes Level 1	20 Minutes Intervals	Rest or Cross Training	20 Minutes Level 1	8 Minutes Hills	20 Minutes x 2 Level 1	30 Minutes Level 1
5	20 Minutes Level 1	10 Minutes Level 2	12 Minutes Level 2	15 Minutes Level 2	20 Minutes Level 2	10 Minutes Hills	35 Minutes Level 1
6	30 Minutes Level 1	20 Minutes x 2 Level 1	20 Minutes x 2 Level 1	Rest or Cross Training	20 Minutes Hills	30 Minutes Intervals	45 Minutes Level 1

Schedule 2 - Beginners

This schedule is designed for beginners in good health but **with only a basic level of fitness**. It's designed to start burning fat from the body's stores and to improve fitness levels so as to progress on to Schedule 3.

The duration and intensity of sessions increase along with fitness levels throughout the course of the 6 weeks.

The sessions are based around level 1 and level 2 walking for the first 4 weeks, but you'll see that there are some more challenging workouts that use hills and interval training principles.

- When performing any hill sessions, you should actually be walking uphill for the stated time, so for example if the schedule lists '5 minutes hills' I want you to walk up a hill or incline for the full 5 minutes.

  This is easily done if you're using a treadmill, but if you're relying on walking up real hills, then you may need to go up and down the same one a few times. Don't rush the downhill part as this is not the aim of the session.

  Unless otherwise written you should walk uphill using level 1 walking speed.

- On any interval sessions throughout Schedule 2, you should use both level 1 and level 2 walking techniques and structure it this way... walk at level 1 for 1 minute and then level 2 for 1 minute and then repeat for the allotted amount of time.

  After week 5, you should also use level 3 walking pace, so this means that you would walk at level 1 for 1 minute, then level 2 for 1 minute and then level 3 for 1 minute. This pattern should be repeated until you have completed the stated time.

- You'll notice throughout the course of the 6 weeks, there are a number of cross training or rest days. This simply means doing nothing or if you feel fine and want to be active then do 30 minutes of an activity other than walking.

- On week 6, there is a Fartlek session, for a full explanation of this have a quick read of the training techniques section. Basically, this is a walking workout where you walk as fast as you can for as far as you can until you feel you need to recover. At which point, you'll slow down until you're ready to go again. You shouldn't stop at any time, instead play around with the speeds that you are walking so you can recover whilst still actually walking.

  Fartlek sessions are more challenging than simply walking and you'll be aiming to get as high as an 8 or 9 on the RPE scale. (See the section on monitoring intensity for more details)

Remember to warm up for 5 minutes before each of the longer or more challenging sessions and then cool down again afterwards for 5 minutes before stretching thoroughly.

If you want to progress from Schedule 2 on to Schedule 3, then I recommend that you complete all of schedule 2 first and then move on to schedule 3.

Schedule 2 – Walking 4 Weight Loss, Beginners Program

WEEKS	MONDAY	TUESDAY	WEDNESDAY	THURSDAY	FRIDAY	SATURDAY	SUNDAY
1	10 Minutes Level 1	10 Minutes Level 1	15 Minutes Level 1	10 Minutes Level 1	10 Minutes Level 1	10 Minutes x 2 Level 1	10 Minutes Level 2
2	15 Minutes Level 1	20 Minutes Level 1	15 Minutes Level 2	10 Minutes Hills	Rest or Cross Training	20 Minutes Level 1	20 Minutes Intervals
3	20 Minutes Level 1	20 Minutes Level 2	20 Minutes Level 1	15 Minutes Hills	Rest or Cross Training	25 Minutes Level 1	30 Minutes Level 1
4	30 Minutes Level 1	25 Minutes Intervals	Rest or Cross Training	30 Minutes Level 2	30 Minutes Level 2	40 Minutes Level 1	60 Minutes Level 1
5	45 Minutes Level 1	Rest or Cross Training	30 Minutes Intervals	35 Minutes Level 2	15 Minutes Level 3	25 Minutes Hills	45 Minutes Level 2
6	20 Minutes Level 3	45 Minutes Intervals	30 Minutes Hills	Rest or Cross Training	60 Minutes Fartlek	35 Minutes Hills	90 Minutes Level 1

Schedule 3 – Active Walker

This schedule is for fit and active people who don't necessarily walk at the moment but do take part in some form of sport or physical activity on a regular basis. It's designed to burn fat quickly from the body's stores and to improve fitness levels.

The duration and intensity of sessions increase along with fitness levels throughout the course of the 8 weeks.

The sessions use all 4 walking levels and also some other challenging walking techniques such as pyramid training, intervals and hill walking to burn off maximum calories whilst minimising impact and keeping workout duration as short as possible.

- When performing any hills sessions, you should actually be walking uphill for the stated time, so for example if the schedule lists '30 minutes hills' I want you to walk up a hill or incline for the majority of the 30 minutes.

  This is easily done if you're using a treadmill, but if you're relying on actually walking up hills, then you may need to go up and down the same one a few times.

  Don't rush the downhill part as this is not the aim of the session, and don't include the time it takes you to walk downhill as part of your workout, because doing so means that you will only end up walking uphill for half the session.

  Unless otherwise written walk uphill using level 2 walking speed throughout schedule 3.

- On any interval sessions throughout Schedule 3, you should use level 1, level 2 and level 3 walking techniques. You can structure this in any way you like, but as an example you could follow this pattern - walk at level 1 for 1 minute and then level 2 for 1 minute and then level 3 for 1 minute. This pattern should be repeated until you have completed the stated time.

- You'll notice throughout the course of the 8 weeks, there are a number of cross training or rest days. This simply means doing 30 minutes of an activity other than walking.

- On weeks 4, 5 and 7 there is a Pyramid session (for a full explanation of this, have a quick read of the training techniques section). You can structure this in any way you like, but as an example throughout a 40 minute Pyramid session, you might walk at level 1 for 5 minutes, then level 2 for 8 minutes, level 3 for 5 minutes and then level 4 for 4 minutes. You've now reached the top of the pyramid and should reduce the level of intensity by walking at level 3 for a further 5 minutes, level 2 for 8 minutes and then 1 for the last 5 minutes to finish with.

  Pyramid sessions should feel more challenging than simply walking and you'll be aiming to get as high as an 8 or 9 on the RPE scale in the middle of your workout before tapering back down again.

Remember to warm up for 5 minutes before each session and then **cool down again afterwards for 5 minutes before stretching thoroughly**. If you want to progress from Schedule 3 on to Schedule 4, then I recommend that you complete all of schedule 3 first and then move on to schedule 4.

Schedule 3 – Walking 4 Weight Loss, Active Persons Program

WEEKS	MONDAY	TUESDAY	WEDNESDAY	THURSDAY	FRIDAY	SATURDAY	SUNDAY
1	20 Minutes x 2 Level 1	20 Minutes x 2 Level 1	30 Minutes Hills	20 Minutes x 2 Level 1	30 Minutes Intervals	20 Minutes x 2 Level 1	60 Minutes Level 1
2	25 Minutes x 2 Level 1	35 Minutes Intervals	20 Minutes x 3 Level 2	25 Minutes x 2 Level 1	45 Minutes x 2 Level 1	35 Minutes Hills	60 Minutes Level 1
3	30 Minutes x 2 Level 1	30 Minutes Level 2	30 Minutes Level 2	Rest or Cross Training	40 Minutes Intervals	30 Minutes x 2 Level 2	70 Minutes Level 1
4	20 Minutes Level 3	40 Minutes Hills	40 Minutes Level 2	Rest or Cross Training	45 Minutes Level 2	40 Minutes Pyramid	75 Minutes Level 1
5	25 Minutes Level 3	45 Minutes Hills	45 Minutes Intervals	20 Minutes x 2 Level 3	60 Minutes Pyramid	Rest or Cross Training	80 Minutes Level 1
6	20 Minutes Hills, Level 3	50 Minutes Intervals	15 Minutes Level 4	20 Minutes Level 4	25 Minutes Hills, Level 3	55 Minutes Intervals	90 Minutes Level 1
7	30 Minutes Hills, Level 3	25 Minutes Level 4	60 Minutes Intervals	Rest or Cross Training	30 Minutes Level 4	60 Minutes Pyramid	100 Minutes Level 1
8	40 Minutes Level 3	60 Minutes Intervals	40 Minutes Level 4	50 Minutes Hills	20 Minutes Hills, Level 4	Rest or Cross Training	120 Minutes Level 1

Schedule 4 – Fit and Wanting a Challenge

This schedule is for very fit people who take part in some form of sport or physical activity on a regular basis and want a higher intensity level of walking. This program really gets going straight away.

It's designed to push the body as hard as possible using walking as the activity of choice. **You should have a good level of fitness before attempting to complete this workout program.** You will burn fat as fast as possible using this training program.

The duration and intensity of sessions increases along with fitness levels throughout the course of the 8 weeks.

The sessions use all 4 walking levels and also some other challenging walking techniques such as pyramid training, intervals, Fartlek and hill walking to burn off maximum calories whilst minimising impact and keeping workouts varied and stimulating. For a full explanation of the various walking levels and advanced techniques see the section on training techniques

- When performing any hills sessions, you should actually be walking uphill for the stated time, so for example if the schedule lists '30 minutes hills' I want you to walk up a hill or incline for the majority of the 30 minutes.

  This is easily done if you're using a treadmill, but if you're relying on actually walking up hills, then you may need to go up and down the same one a few times.

  Don't rush the downhill part as this is not the aim of the session, and don't include the time it takes you to walk downhill as part of your workout, because doing so means that you will only end up walking uphill for half the session.

Unless otherwise written you should walk uphill on your hill sessions using level 2 walking speed throughout schedule 4.

- On any interval sessions throughout Schedule 4, you can structure them in any way you like, but as an example you should use all levels of walking technique like this - walk at level 1 for 1 minute, then level 2 for 1 minute, then level 3 for 1 minute and finally level 4 for 1 minute. This pattern should be repeated until you have completed the stated time.

- You'll notice throughout the course of the 8 weeks, there are several cross training or rest days. This simply means doing nothing or if you feel fine and want to be active then do 30 – 60 minutes of an activity other than walking.

- On weeks 2, 4, 5 and 8 there is a Pyramid session. Basically, this is a walking workout where you begin by walking at level 1 and build up to level 4 in the middle of the session.

- You can structure this in any way you like, but as an example throughout a 40 minute Pyramid session, you might walk at level 1 for 5 minutes, then level 2 for 8 minutes, level 3 for 5 minutes and then level 4 for 4 minutes. You've now reached the top of the pyramid and should begin to reduce the level of intensity by walking at level 3 for a further 5 minutes, level 2 for 8 minutes and then 1 for the last 5 minutes to finish with.

- Pyramid sessions should feel more challenging than simply walking and you'll be aiming to get as high as an 8 or 9 on the RPE scale in the middle of your workout before tapering back down again.

- On weeks 4, 6 and 7 there are Fartlek sessions. Fartlek training is basically a walking workout where you walk as fast as you can for as far as you can until you feel you need to recover. At which point, you'll slow down until you're ready to go again.

You shouldn't stop at any time, instead play around with the speeds that you are walking at so you can recover whilst still actually walking. Fartlek sessions should feel more challenging than simply walking along and you'll be aiming to get as high as an 8 or 9 on the RPE scale.

Remember to warm up for 5 minutes before each session and then cool down again afterwards for 5 minutes before stretching thoroughly.

Schedule 4 – Walking 4 Weight Loss, Very Fit Persons Program

WEEKS	MONDAY	TUESDAY	WEDNESDAY	THURSDAY	FRIDAY	SATURDAY	SUNDAY
1	30 Minutes x 2 Level 2	45 Minutes Level 1	Rest or Cross Training	45 Minutes Intervals	30 Minutes Hills	20 Minutes Level 3	45 Minutes Level 2
2	25 Minutes Level 3	50 Minutes Intervals	Rest or Cross Training	25 Minutes x 2 Level 3	30 Minutes Fartlek	30 Minutes Pyramid	50 Minutes Level 2
3	30 Minutes Hills, Level 2	30 Minutes Level 3	Rest or Cross Training	35 Minutes Level 3	50 Minutes Intervals	Rest or Cross Training	55 Minutes Level 2
4	40 Minutes Level 3	40 Minutes Hills, Level 2	Rest or Cross Training	40 Minutes Pyramid	45 Minutes Level 3	35 Minutes Fartlek	60 Minutes Level 2
5	20 Minutes Level 4	45 Minutes Fartlek	Rest or Cross Training	50 Minutes Pyramid	20 Minutes Hills, Level 3	15 Minutes x 2 Level 4	65 Minutes Level 2
6	30 Minutes Hills, Level 3	55 Minutes Intervals	Rest or Cross Training	25 Minutes Level 4	25 Minutes Hills, Level 4	50 Minutes Fartlek	70 Minutes Level 2
7	40 Minutes Hills, Level 3	30 Minutes Level 4	Rest or Cross Training	55 Minutes Intervals	35 Minutes Hills, Level 4	60 Minutes Fartlek	75 Minutes Level 2
8	40 Minutes Level 4	60 Minutes Intervals	Rest or Cross Training	60 Minutes Pyramid	45 Minutes Hills, Level 4	50 Minutes Level 4	80 Minutes Level 2

Schedule 5 - Maintenance

When you've made it this far, you'll have reached your weight loss goals and simply need to maintain your success. This schedule is designed to continue using some of the techniques you've learnt over the past few weeks and to maintain a good level of fitness at the same time.

The sessions use all 4 walking levels and also some other challenging walking techniques such as pyramid training, intervals, hill walking and Fartlek training to burn off maximum calories whilst minimising impact and keeping workout duration as short as possible.

- When performing any hills sessions, you should be walking uphill for the stated period of time, so for example if the schedule lists '30 minutes hills,' I want you to actually be walking up a hill or incline for the majority of the 30 minutes. This is easily done if you're using a treadmill, but if you're relying on walking up actual hills, then you may need to go up and down the same one a few times.

   Don't rush the downhill part as this is not the aim of the session, and don't include the time it takes you to walk downhill as part of your workout, because doing so means that you will only end up walking uphill for half the session. Unless otherwise written you should walk uphill using level 2 walking speed throughout schedule 5.

- On any interval sessions throughout Schedule 5, you should use all of the different walking levels and structure it this way... walk at level 1 for 1 minute, level 2 for 1 minute, then level 3 for 1 minute and finally level 4 for 1 minute. Repeat until you have completed the time.

- You'll notice throughout the course of the 6 weeks, there are a few cross training days. This simply means doing another activity other than walking.

- On Pyramid sessions, begin by walking at level 1 and build up to level 4 in the middle of the session. You can structure this in any way you like, but as an example throughout a 40 minute Pyramid session, you might walk at level 1 for 5 minutes, then level 2 for 8 minutes, level 3 for 5 minutes and then level 4 for 4 minutes. You've now reached the top of the pyramid and should begin to reduce the level of intensity by walking at level 3 for a further 5 minutes, level 2 for 8 minutes and then 1 for the last 5 minutes to finish with.

Pyramid sessions are more challenging than simply walking and you'll be aiming to get as high as an 8 or 9 on the RPE scale in the middle of your workout before tapering down.

- On week 4 there is a Fartlek session. Fartlek training is basically a walking workout where you walk as fast as you can for as far as you can until you feel you need to recover. At which point, you'll slow down until you're ready to go again.

You shouldn't stop at any time, instead play around with the speeds that you are walking at so you can recover whilst still actually walking. Fartlek sessions should feel more challenging than simply walking along and you'll be aiming to get as high as an 8 or 9 on the RPE scale.

Remember to warm up for 5 minutes before each session and then **cool down again afterwards before stretching thoroughly**.

Schedule 5 – Walking 4 Weight Loss, Maintenance Program

WEEKS	MONDAY	TUESDAY	WEDNESDAY	THURSDAY	FRIDAY	SATURDAY	SUNDAY
1	20 Minutes x 2 Level 2	Cross Training 45 Minutes	25 Minutes Hills, Level 2	Rest	30 Minutes Level 3	Cross Training 30 Minutes	60 Minutes Level 2
2	20 Minutes x 2 Level 3	Cross Training 40 Minutes	30 Minutes Intervals	Rest	30 Minutes Level 4	Cross Training 40 Minutes	60 Minutes Level 2
3	20 Minutes x 2 Level 4	Cross Training 30 Minutes	30 Minutes Pyramid	Rest	35 Minutes Hills	Cross Training 30 Minutes	90 Minutes Level 1
4	30 Minutes x 2 Level 2	Cross Training 45 Minutes	60 Minutes Fartlek	Rest	60 Minutes Pyramid	Cross Training 40 Minutes	60 Minutes Level 2
5	30 Minutes x 2 Level 3	Cross Training 40 Minutes	60 Minutes Level 3	Rest	60 Minutes Intervals	Cross Training 30 Minutes	90 Minutes Level 1
6	30 Minutes x 2 Level 4	Cross Training 30 Minutes	60 Minutes Hills, Level 3	Rest	30 Minutes Level 4	Cross Training 40 Minutes	60 Minutes Level 2

Active Living Tips

AIM TO DO AT LEAST ONE SESSION OF ACTIVITY/EXERCISE PER DAY. Set some time aside at the beginning of the week to plan the activities you intend to do.

The following forms of activities are some that could be included: - Heavy gardening, cleaning all the windows in the house, walking up and down the steps a certain number of times in an hour etc.

Why not plan a few different walking routes which include a few hills and inclines.

Find out if there are any structured fitness classes you could start attending locally.

AIM TO GET SWEATY WHILST EXERCISING. With this type of bodily response you can be confident that your heart and lungs are working sufficiently hard to promote effective fat burning.

PARK THE CAR FURTHER AWAY FROM WORK. By doing this you are forcing yourself to be more active and get more exercise. If you catch the bus, why not get off one or two stops earlier or better still walk the whole way to work if possible.

AVOID USING ESCALAORS OR THE LIFT. Instead take the stairs.

START YOUR NEW REGIME WITH A FRIEND. By starting upon a fitness programme with a friend you ensure a number of things happen: -

- They will experience the same sensations of exercise as you which will make it easier and more sociable.
- There will be support and motivation between you both.
- You will be able to encourage and provide each other with a sounding board and a willing listener.
- You will have someone to share your success who knows the effort you are putting in.
- WHEN WALKING MAKE A CONSCIOUS EFFORT TO INCREASE THE SPEED. Even when you are simply strolling aim to increase your speed which in effect will burn off more calories.
- WHEN SHOPPING PARK AT THE FURTHEST POINT. By parking at the furthest point from the supermarket door again you ensure that you are performing more exercise than you would have otherwise done.
- PULL YOUSELF TOGETHER. If your job involves a lot of sitting down or you sit a lot in the evenings try to pull yourself up straighter instead of slouching and reclining...

Sit with your stomach muscles pulled in tight (Don't hold your breath) and shoulders back and back straight.

Aim to increase the length of time you can do this for without feeling uncomfortable. You will be surprised how short an amount of time this will be to begin with.

LEAVE THE REMOTE CONTROL BY THE TV. By manually changing the channels on the TV or setting the video it has been found that the average person could lose one pound of body fat each year.

Surprising the effects a little effort can have!

CLEAN THE CAR AND WAX IT. Don't you find cleaning and waxing the car hard work... I do.

Imagine how popular you'll be if this job gets done at least once a week and think about the calories you are burning.

The suggestions above are by no means exhaustive and have been added to give an indication of what active living is all about. For example, these days most TV's can't be changed manually, but hopefully you get the picture. A small change can bring about surprisingly big results over time.

Prehistoric men and women had to hunt and live in stone huts foraging for firewood and food. The very nature of this existence meant that obesity and lack of exercise was rare.

These days we need to introduce activities and exercise to encourage healthy living to offset the effects of inactivity. We were not designed to be a sedentary species and many of today's degenerative illness can be attributed to poor diet and lack of exercise.

Final Thoughts

I hope you've enjoyed reading my walking manual and that you've learnt something, but more importantly that *you feel motivated and ready to take action*. Action is where it all starts.

Here a quick recap of what you need to do next...

1. If you have any health or injury issues or concerns or are over the age of 50, I suggest a quick visit to your doctor or physician to get a check-up.

2. Get your pen and paper out, you're going to start doing some planning. **Planning and recording are one of the most undervalued parts of the entire process of change.** Once you record what you're planning to do, your goals and targets etc, it will become more than just a thought.

Once you've committed your goals to paper, they become a useful tool. **Keep them in a prominent position** so you can see them and keep motivated, rewrite them if necessary as you progress.

3. If you need some new footwear, then get these next.

4. Look at your diet and make sure you are making the changes needed to see a reduction in your weight. If you follow one of the walking programs and **reduce your daily intake by 200 - 300kcals** then you should be on track to lose at least 1lb a week. This is easily done if you look for any high calorie snacks you eat and cut them out of your diet.

5. Read through the various walking programs to decide which one you should start with and then plan in your diary for the days and times you'll do your walking sessions.

6. **Take some photos and measurements of your weight, hips and waist and record these**.

Before you start, please remember that Rome wasn't built in a day. If you want to use walking to get into great shape you need to be consistent and do the right things most of the time.

It's fine to have the occasional treat and rest day, just don't let it become a regular habit that gradually takes over your life again.

Any fitness benefits will stop if you stop exercising. There's an old saying in the fitness industry which simply goes '*use it or lose it*.' Any improvements in muscle tone, body shape, fitness levels etc will gradually deteriorate after you stop exercising, which can happen in weeks, so stay active.

Finally, TO GET THE BEST OUT OF THIS SYSTEM YOU ABSOLUTELY HAVE LOOK AT THE WAY YOU EAT. If your goal is weight loss, then you'll become very de-motivated if you don't make changes to your diet. Small changes will be enough at first to see real improvements, but if you want to get into amazing shape you'll need to work on your diet so it's consistently very good.

I wish you every success with your walking, please let me know how you get on by sending me an email here – jago@anewimage.co.uk

Warmest regards

Jago

Other Books That Might Be of Interest to You...

Here are a couple of great recipe books which will help to keep you energised and feeling wonderful all day long. You'll discover loads of delicious recipes which are low in fat, easy to make and use relatively inexpensive ingredients. Click on the blue text links below to find out more and discover a wonderful collection of some of the tastiest salad and soups recipes around!

Healthy Soups

Today's fast pace of life and our busy lifestyles means that many of us simply don't eat the right types of foods. We forget to eat or don't have the time, so instead we eat on the run and make poor food choices which lead to weight gain and a lack of energy.

Not only do many of us eat the wrong kinds of food in the first place, but we also neglect to eat enough of the good things. Well, here's your chance to put things right, with over 50 of the tastiest juicing recipes which are easy to make and packed full of goodness:

https://www.amazon.com/dp/B00A8I9PRI

Healthy Salads

Preparing your own healthy food often means slaving away for hours; but most of the super quick salads and dressings in this book can be prepared and ready to eat in less than 10 minutes!

Another great thing about making your own salad is that it can be a very cheap meal for anyone cooking on a budget. Salads are no longer simply a summer dish, with some of the warm salads in this book you can also treat yourself to a healthy, warming and refreshing meal in the middle of winter:

https://www.amazon.com/dp/B009FT4PFI

5K Training for Beginners

Many people struggle to fit a time for exercise into their busy lifestyles- and it's an understandable problem. You've got to have time to spare. You need to get to the gym, get changed, do your workout, get showered and changed again and then travel back home. Depending on where you live and your work schedule, this could so easily take up a couple of hours of your precious time.

But there is a solution... Running, but not running as you know it. Go here to find out more about a unique running system you can start today:

https://www.amazon.com/dp/B0085VG410

Aims and Objectives

Four Week / Short Term Aims

AIM #1
AIM #2
AIM #3
AIM #4

To Achieve This I Will : -

Twelve Week / Mid Term Aims

AIM #1
AIM #2
AIM #3
AIM #4

To Achieve This I Will : -

Long Term Aims

AIM #1
AIM #2
AIM #3
AIM #4

To Achieve This I Will : -

Weekly Measurements

How to use this form

Whenever you set out on a journey it is important that you chart your progress regularly. Jumping on the scales every day certainly isn't productive, but I would recommend that you do this once a week and take your measurements at the same time.

You should use your hips and waist measurements and not your weight to assess whether or not progress is being made. By taking measurements at regular intervals you are doing 2 things. Firstly you can see whether your current efforts are having effect, if they are keep doing what you are doing, if not make some changes. For example you might be able to increase the amount of activity you are doing.

Secondly it maintains your awareness and helps to keep you focused on your goals and objectives.

Date	Weight	Waist	Hips

Start your measurements on week 1. Take them at the same time and day each week. Measure around the narrowest part of your waist and the widest part of your hips.

Your Workout Log

Date:	Training Time:	Day:
Vital Statistics		
Resting Heart Rate Before:		
Weight:		
Sleep in Hours, Night Before:		
Eaten Well Through the Day:		
Workout Type:	Overall Difficulty Level (1-10):	
Distance:		
Course:		
Duration:		
Average Heart Rate:	End Heart Rate:	
Weather:	Temperature:	
Mood and Enjoyment		
Hated it:		
Felt Great:		
Really Enjoyed it:		
Was OK:		
Notes:		

You can use this form to monitor your workouts and chart your progress. You may want to use all the sections in the form or just a few. Whatever you do decide, just make sure that you have a record of your sessions. This will help motivate you to do more in the future and perhaps more importantly reinforce the fact that what you've done in the past is helping you to get fitter.

I suggest that you copy this page and print one out for each session you do.

Activity Planner

WEEKS	MONDAY	TUESDAY	WEDNESDAY	THURSDAY	FRIDAY	SATURDAY	SUNDAY
1							
2							
3							
4							

Plan your activities in advance, choose things you enjoy. Aim to do some form of activity at least 5 times a week.

Printed in Great Britain
by Amazon

37054308R00071